WHERE'S MY PURSE?

T. A. SORENSEN

ISBN-10: 1499370806
ISBN-13: 9781499370805

DEDICATION

To JoAnn
My Mother, Best Friend, Hero.
I Love You.

ACKNOWLEDGMENTS

There are no words powerful enough to express how grateful I am to my mother's caregivers. The patience, love and nurturing they exhibit is unmatched. To encounter and manage what they do, each and every day, requires a character rich in strength and compassion. I would like to thank them, from the bottom of my heart.

My contributors are also a brave group of individuals. The only way one can fully understand how it feels to sit in their boots, is to experience dealing with Alzheimer's first-hand. Each of them generously opened up and shared very personal moments through their stories. I'm incredibly grateful for their trust and their contributions.

I would also like to thank my editor, Patricia, for her kindness and patience. I'm honored that she accepted my project and became my friend during the process.

Thank you to Karen Tawater, the brilliant individual who photographed the cover of my book.

The Alzheimer's Association allowed me to reference facts, when warranted, from articles posted to their website and for that, I am very appreciative.

CONTENTS

Acknowledgments V

PART ONE - REMINISCENCE

    Foreword 3
1   JoAnn 5
2   A Little "Skippy" 13
3   Funk Is In The Air. 21
4   Home Sweet "Home". 25
5   Resuming. 31
6   W-T-F 35
7   The Little Bitches That Clean 39
8   And You Are?. 45
9   Part I: In Search Of 53
10   Part II: In Search Of. 59
11   Red Flags Abound 63
12   Breaking Mom. 73
13   Tour De Nécessité 81
14   A Perfect Fit. 89
15   Before The Well Runs Dry 97
16   Seven 101
17   Perspectives 109

18   Where's My Purse?. 113

      Epilogue. 117

PART TWO - RECOLLECTION

19   Christine 121

20   Pop. 129

21   Albert. 137

22   Ernie. 145

23   Isabelle. 149

24   Life With Larry 159

      About The Author. 183

PART ONE

REMINISCENCE

FOREWORD

If you're wondering why I am embarking on this project, it's simple. I'm losing my mother, my best friend, to this malady called Alzheimer's and I'm pissed! Watching someone you love change so drastically can be an incredibly painful and frustrating process. One moment you're engaging in a "normal" dialogue with them and the next, they're sharing a story with you about an event that never took place. Their Walter Mitty-esque reality is mind-boggling.

Eventually, the dance becomes very tedious and you find yourself becoming frustrated and resentful. Stepping back and looking at the big picture, I made a conscious choice to alter my perspective, and view what is "right" with my mother's world, instead of focusing on what "I" am experiencing. I made a vow to always make it about her and ensure that she is happy and cared for. There will be plenty of time for self-pity after my mother is gone.

When this journey began, I started researching, as one does. There was a plethora of material available based on facts and figures, but it wasn't enough. What I needed, was a truthful, first-hand account from someone walking the same road, which would provide me with some sense of what lay ahead. My sincere hope in writing the following story is that by sharing what I deem to be my raw, private, family moments, I might be able to comfort someone else.

So please indulge me, while I furnish you with a little back history on my Mom. And keep in mind that everything I share will make sense, as you progress through the book.

Welcome to my journey.

———⟨⟨⟨⟩⟩⟩———

JOANN

JoAnn was born in Anaconda, Montana, circa 1929, to John and Winnie Floy. Her father worked as a commercial bus driver, while her mother perfected her role as a Southern Belle. When Mom reached the ripe old age of twelve, her sister "Punky" was born. Unfortunately, Winnie passed away shortly thereafter, and JoAnn instantly added the role of Pseudo-Mommy to her CV. One thing about Mom has remained consistent to this day: she has always loved her family more than life and would do anything for them.

During her high school years, she was a cheerleader and ran with, in her words, "the kids from the other side of the tracks." A privileged child who didn't fashion herself as "entitled"; everyone was on equal footing with her. As long as you possessed a sense of humor and were able to make her laugh, you were invited into her world. She was loyal, witty, smart, and a bit naughty, always ending up as the center of attention, but never intentionally seeking it.

In 1948, she married Bob, whom she dated in high school. They moved to Oregon, then eventually to Seattle, where they would permanently reside. Mom became a nurse and worked very hard, to support herself and my father until he finished Dental school. He set up a thriving practice and together, they produced three children - two daughters and a son - who were truly the loves of her life. Bob's fifteen years of infidelity led to their divorce in 1972.

My recurring memories of Mom always include her white smile, red lips and equally as red fingernails, which I still affectionately refer to as her "talons." She smelled of Emeraude perfume and her hair was perfectly in place. Her car of choice, a Cadillac; the last one a black model with fins, nicknamed the "Hearse" by our friends. We lived in an area where everyone knew each other and attended one of two grade schools. If the "Hearse" was spotted outside of our school building prior to 3:15 p.m., one of us was in trouble, and a challenging evening lay ahead.

Silly as it may sound, that car represented security and love to me. I didn't care that it was a luxury automobile - I cared that it was parked outside, by the playground, waiting for me every day without fail.

JoAnn was a loving disciplinarian with a strict regimen, to which we were held accountable. Pitching in with laundry, housekeeping and meals was expected. Each Saturday she would enter our rooms, throw our shutters open no later than 7:30 a.m. and announce to us that it was time to get up. "Move your bones! This is going to be a busy day for you and as soon as all of the weeding is done, we can spend time together," was the Saturday proclamation. We'd comply, and after breakfast the three of us would head outdoors into the garden to start.

In an effort to encourage her hard working crew, she purchased each one of us our own tiny bucket, hand claw, shovel, and pair of gloves. Lunch was always delivered on the back porch at 12:00 p.m. sharp, and three dimes were brought out a few hours later in anticipation of the ice cream truck motoring past. When the work was complete, we would head in for a bath and supper. But before we sat down for our meal, we would go back outside together, holding hands in a line to review our efforts. On cue, Mom would exclaim how beautiful everything looked and reinforce how much she appreciated our help. I can still recall beaming with pride.

Holidays in our home were extremely special. The moment we spied Santa aboard the Norelco shaver in the TV commercial, the decorations came down from the attic. A bit of a perfectionist, she preferred to handle the décor on the main tree herself; however, we were her assembly team. She'd light a fire, turn on Rudolph and bring out cups of hot cocoa with giant marshmallows. The artificial tree limbs were dumped out of the box and placed on the living room floor so we could group them by their color-coded tips. Once the tree was assembled, she would carry various boxes of ornaments downstairs, where a live tree awaited our touch. By the time the three of us were finished, the tree could barely be seen through the tinsel. But, forever our champion, she would wade through the sea of broken bulbs and begin praising our masterpiece as though it was the most beautiful tree she had ever seen.

JoAnn's playful side was another wonderful attribute worth mentioning. I remember one evening, while she was preparing dinner, she asked all three of us to sit quietly in front of the refrigerator, and if we could be silent for an entire three minutes, she would give each of us a shiny nickel. We immediately huddled together, watching the second hand intently, when all of a sudden she broke into song, began to dance, and flipped her dental bridge out to expose bare gums. Needless to say, no money exchanged hands.

Labeling Mom a "Clotheshorse" would be a gross understatement. When I was growing up, every closet in our home had a large, square, cloth storage bag in it filled with her clothes. Amongst my most special memories are the times I sat on the floor in my parents' bathroom visiting with Mom, while she readied herself for an evening engagement. The stunning gowns she would retrieve from the upstairs closet, the elbow-length gloves adorned with various cocktail rings, her drop earrings, beaded evening bag and shoes to match; she was the most beautiful woman I had ever seen.

During my youth, I often felt out of place with other kids because when they were complaining about their mothers, I had zero to contribute. Spending time with my family was my preference. True, Mom was very strict, but she provided a sense of security that a lot of my friends craved. I suppose that's why our home was like Grand Central Station; always full of laughter, friends and most importantly, love. We were very blessed.

Strength was another attribute that JoAnn possessed and it was certainly tested when my sister, Tamara, was diagnosed with Acute Myelogenous Leukemia, or AML, two weeks prior to her Sweet Sixteen. Mom was raising three children on her own and now one of them was going to be hospitalized for God knows how long, provided she survived. A difficult, but necessary decision was made to send both my brother and me to stay with our Godparents, making it possible for Mom to move into a small, cubicle-sized room outside of my sister's room at the hospital. We were safe, well cared for, and JoAnn was exactly where she needed to be.

My sister required many blood transfusions, so the three of us worked in rotation. Because JoAnn was a constant fixture at the hospital and Tamara was requiring so many transfusions, Mom opted to have a shunt implanted into her forearm, which would enable her to donate blood at a moment's notice. One afternoon, while being hooked up to the machines for the extraction, an incident took place in which a blood clot escaped from the shunt into Mom's bloodstream. This resulted in her experiencing a mild stroke. She has always kept that information from my sister and almost everyone else, but me. I didn't understand why she didn't want anyone to know at the time, but I do now. It was an unfortunate incident, but she was fine and getting Tamara well was her only focus. Her priorities were always in order; she never needed a pat on the back, or the applause.

The battle against the disease was finally won. Following a successful bone marrow transplant, radiation treatments, chemotherapy and every side effect known to man, my sister was deemed cured. Her physician at the time, Dr. E. Donnell Thomas, was awarded the Nobel Prize for Medicine in 1990. Dr. Thomas was responsible for developing bone marrow transplantation as a treatment for leukemia, which ultimately saved my sister's life.

The few memories about Mom I've singled out in this chapter don't even scratch the surface. In my Foreword, I asked the reader to "indulge me" because I felt it was important to provide some sense of who JoAnn is at her core, as opposed to how she currently presents, with Alzheimer's. If I were asked to describe her before AD using only adjectives, I would say: vibrant, active, athletic, caring, loving, funny, silly, artistic, spiritual, intelligent, wise, loyal and beautiful. Now, albeit she is no longer as mobile (or noisy), if you look very closely into her eyes, the same descriptors would apply.

A LITTLE "SKIPPY"

In 1978, Mom got remarried to a man named Jim. They had known each other since high school, where they shared a mutual infatuation. Despite that mild flirtation, their paths led them in different directions, until one fall day, many years later, they were reunited. Jim served as a Captain in the Navy, and following their wedding, his tour of duty took them to California, Okinawa, and finally back to Washington, where they enjoyed their retirement. Aside from the birth of her children, the day she married him was her happiest.

Fast-forward to Christmas evening of 2006. Jim became very ill during dinner and, as the night progressed, his condition worsened. Because they lived 2½ hours northwest of a trauma center, he had to be airlifted to Seattle. He was admitted to the ICU and placed on a respirator. In a matter of hours, Jim had slipped into renal failure and soon after, a coma. He remained in that state for three months, which marked the beginning of Mom's journey with Alzheimer's disease.

If you've ever visited an Intensive Care Unit, you've no doubt noticed that there are very small, private waiting areas, where family members spend the majority of their time. Brought together under adverse circumstances, they become each other's support system and extended family. One morning, I was pulled aside for a chat by a woman whose husband was also in the ICU. Visibly uncomfortable, she expressed a genuine concern for my mom. Apparently, JoAnn was repeating herself and sharing the same stories, over and over. In Mom's defense, I told the lady that my mom was tired and stressed out. Truth be told, I knew an issue existed and it was being exacerbated by the circumstances. The issue with her repeating herself had been going on for several months and each time we addressed it, the blanket response would be, "I'm just a little skippy." Knowing that two of her relatives had been diagnosed with Alzheimer's disease, it only made sense to explore this further.

Later that evening, I asked Mom to go for a walk. Arm-in-arm, we cruised around the hallways of the hospital, stepping into the gift shop for a peek, anything to stall. Finally, we retired to a couple of chairs away from everyone, and I asked her if she would do me a favor. "Sure, anything," was her reply. Taking both of her hands in mine and declaring how much I loved her, I voiced my concerns, asking if she would humor me by having a checkup. Again, her explanation was, "I'm just a little skippy." Expressing as gently as possible that it seemed to be more than "skippy", JoAnn agreed to consider an exam.

Fortunately for all, my stepfather, Jim, recovered and came home. But life was never going to be the same. The dialog Mom and I shared during our walk, three weeks prior, must have struck a chord with her. Unbeknownst to me, she did see a physician and her fears were realized. The call came to me about 8:30 p.m. one evening and I answered to the sound of Mom's sobbing; "You were right. He said you were right. I have Alzheimer's." There is no way one can prepare for this type of call, and, as you might expect, my heart was crushed.

I'm a "fixer" by nature, so wrapping my head around this new revelation along with the knowledge that I was powerless to fix it, was a tough pill to swallow. At a minimum, I needed to attempt to comfort my mom in a meaningful way. So, I sat down, put pen to paper and showed her my heart in a good old fashioned letter, which read:

"To My Friend ~

I felt this card was extremely appropriate and everything it says is exactly how I feel. Also this letter is long over-due. On those days you feel confused and empty, I want you to pick it up and read it again.

Over the past couple of years, I've witnessed the same woman that I grew up admiring, rise to the occasion so many times. From Jim's illness to the nasty hand you've been dealt with your health, you never miss a beat. Irrespective of the fact that you have been saddled with an awful disease, you remain, ever the caretaker, for your husband, your children, your friends.

When I told you that I refused to baby you, I meant it! I make it a policy to always put myself in the other person's place and I wouldn't want to be treated as though I were mindless and incapable of making decisions. I'd be in-sulted. My guarantee to you is that it won't happen with me. You have always been my heroine, my rock and will remain so.

Vivid memories of my childhood are with me each and every day and totally explain why I turned out like this!

Of Bob - The arguments, the loud voices through my bedroom wall, the crying, the swearing, your black eye, being tossed a toy upon his arrival at home, when he yet again, missed dinner, his grapefruit slices in the glass container, Tiger's milk with pineapple juice, his gray

*gym bag, the hair net, cigarettes in his Chevy along-
side deerskin driving gloves, his vulgar comments to
me in front of his office staff, while having me literally
picked up and thrown out onto the sidewalk outside of
his office.*

*Of You – Combing Trux' hair with the green goop, fak-
ing like you were crying to get us to scratch your legs
and rub your feet, while you sat in your gold chair,
screaming when we placed raw creepy crawlers in your
bed, just to make us laugh, paying us to not say a word
for five minutes and then flipping out your bridge to
again, make us laugh, playing in the pool with us,
hot cocoa waiting for us on our desks after school, for
Valentine's Day you had stuffed animals and candy
on our beds when we got home – even in high school,
decorating the Christmas tree after assembling it, playing Chutes and Ladders and Monopoly with us, dy-
ing eggs at Easter, throwing great parties, making us
fudge on weekends, making us hamburgers for lunch
and dropping us at the ski bus every Saturday, break-
fasts at the Barb after Mass each Sunday, picking us
up in the black Cadillac (the Hearse), taking us out
to see how nice the yard looked, once the gardens were
weeded (by us), always attending our sporting activities and yelling the loudest, sticking up for me when
the school called to say I was missing in action, giving me the opportunity to confess later on that I had
skipped school and actually listening to my explanation, your gowns and matching accessories, your braid
in the right-hand bathroom drawer, your Emeraude*

powder, you listening to us when we needed an ear and offering your advice albeit unsolicited and supporting me through my many missteps.

The list could go on for days, but by now, you get the picture. The common theme throughout this list of memories I have of you is that you were always with us and for us. You made our lives secure and happy, despite the circumstances and continue to be our anchor, although we'd like to believe we're completely out of the nest. I'm pissed that you were diagnosed with Alzheimer's disease. I don't understand how this could happen to such a wonderful, selfless person. The selfish side of me doesn't want to lose you, but I'm mostly angry for you. I can't know how you feel, I can only imagine. Hopefully, you'll allow me to be a source of comfort and strength for you, just as you have been for me. Be confident that I would do anything for you.

Thank you for being my Mom and truly becoming my friend. From my pharmaceutical "experiments" and stream of bad calls with respect to men, you've always glued yourself into my corner. You afforded me the freedom to develop a mind of my own and respected my choices, even though at times, they were in direct conflict with your beliefs. Bottom line, you accept and love me without conditions, but most importantly, you've taught me how to love properly.

I admire you, respect you and love you deeply.

Tary"

She never mentioned receiving the letter, but when I was cleaning out Jim and Mom's home, I found it tucked into the back corner of her linen closet, alongside all of the other cards I had sent her prior to that day.

FUNK IS IN THE AIR

Anyone who knew my mom was aware of her housekeeping standards. You've heard the old adage "The floor was so clean, you could eat off of it." Well in our home, that probably wasn't far from the truth. The moment you walked in, the waft of scented candles permeated the air. Every room was spotless and tidy, the cupboards perfectly organized and the inside of the refrigerator looked like an advertisement. That is until Alzheimer's came into play.

My husband Dean and I cherished the time we spent with my parents. We vacationed with them and spent numerous weekends at their home enjoying golf outings. As we hadn't been up in approximately four weeks, we decided to head to their house early one Saturday morning for a visit. Upon entering the front door, something was distinctly off. There was a strange funk in the air that I couldn't identify, but it was pungent! A search ensued to locate the source and the discovery was unsettling.

The inside of the refrigerator had become a gigantic petri dish, housing a vast array of bacterial experiments. Leftovers uncovered, expired dairy products, rotten vegetables, old take-out boxes, you name it and incorporate mold, it was there. My husband grabbed the largest black garbage bags he could find and held them open for me, while I discarded the rotting groceries. Moving on to the cupboards, we encountered a bag of spoiled and leaking potatoes, open boxes of cereal and a bevy of items that should have been refrigerated. The trash compactor had not been cleaned and was spilling over. Taking a step back, once we were finished, Dean and I glanced around the room; there sat eight giant garbage bags filled to the brim. How on earth could I have missed the signs? This event left me speechless.

Fearing this was only the beginning, I moved down the hallway to inspect the first bathroom and was sickened. Fully aware Mom had Alzheimer's disease, there was still a tiny piece of her little girl that hoped it would pass. Reality settled in, and I knew at that very moment it was now my turn to take care of her, and our roles had permanently reversed. I grabbed some gloves along with a can of cleanser, and no sooner did the sponge hit the inside of the bowl, when in walked Mom. She inquired as to what I was doing, and immediately burst into tears. My initial instinct was to throw my arms around her and halt the cleaning. Instead, I told her she was being silly and stated, "There's nothing wrong with a little help, now and again." The lump in my throat was the size of a walnut.

I finished cleaning the remainder of the up-stairs, while my husband, Dean, ran the vacuum. Executing a quick once-over of the laundry room, I observed that the ironing basket was empty and the wash had been kept up. Interesting; you can't smell rotting food, but your clothes are clean and ironed. Welcome to the new thought process!

We decided to run down to the store and pur-chase some groceries, so I could prepare dinner for everyone. Following our meal, the leftovers, along with a few additional items, were packaged, labeled and placed in my parents' freezer. The cleaning was never spoken of again, but on my way out, Mom whispered "Thank you" in my ear, while hugging and kissing me, and frankly, that padded my heart a bit.

Phoning to check on her was nothing out of the ordinary. In fact, she was my best friend and we'd often share a cocktail over the phone on Saturday evenings. But after this particular weekend, all of my senses were on high alert and I thought it best to follow up. Strategically selecting a time when she would normally be in the middle of her dinner preparation, I called her up. Understand that this woman was organized; everything in her life was scheduled like clockwork. As suspected, the supper prep was not happening. Gently, I reminded her of the dinners that we packaged for them and suggested she go look in the freezer while I waited. Several minutes later, JoAnn returned to the phone with a packet of frozen string beans. We worked together for fifteen minutes to thaw out the legumes, during which I provided her a refresher course on Microwave 101. It became blatantly clear that Assisted Living was going to be the next step.

HOME SWEET "HOME"

The search for an Assisted Living facility is grueling, but not nearly as painful as convincing your parents to move into one. I suppose it's understandable, given that up until this juncture, they've been self-sufficient. In explaining to them that it's in their best interest, the only thing they hear is, "You are incompetent." My situation was no exception.

Following dozens of phone interviews and equally as many tours, I finally located the perfect Assisted Living facility, approximately two miles from their home. The thought was that they would still be on familiar turf and remain in close proximity to their friends. Both were extremely resistant. Mom had no recollection that she had even toured the building and Dad, being a retired naval officer and male, had not come to terms with the fact that he needed help. My favorite way to describe the process: It was like trying to coax two feral cats into a carrier.

Jim's health post-coma, never quite returned to normal. Diagnosed with COPD (Chronic Obstructive Pulmonary Disease) and Congestive Heart, he was required to intake oxygen fulltime. Because the oxygen tank was yet another reminder that he needed assistance, he would leave it in the car when they went out. The third time I was summoned for the 2¾ hour drive to the hospital because he had again collapsed on the sidewalk, I sat on the edge of his bed and furnished him with a couple of options. He could put his ego aside and move into the facility that I had found, or he could take my number out of his phone and find someone else to come to his aid the next time it happened. Don't misunderstand me; he was a very loving man, a great partner to my mom, and I loved him as if he were my own father. But, he was no longer strong enough to handle the day-to-day, let alone what lay ahead. In the end, he agreed and relieved, I cried the entire way home. Tough love sucks!

We chose not to share the news about moving with Mom quite yet, as she was still very resistant, as well as concerned that we were trying to take her home away. In reality, our only intention was to protect her. The well-orchestrated moving day arrived, and Mom's wonderful girlfriend arranged to pick her up for a shopping trip. The moment they left the house, we got to work. Our team of five sorted through Jim and JoAnn's possessions, taking only what we felt they actually needed. Endeavoring to make the transition smooth, we configured the new apartment to appear as a mirror image of their home. Custom drapes were installed, including the valances, the area rugs were placed appropriately, and the wall art was hung.

My mother was in the early stages at this point, so I am guessing that when they drove up to the large Assisted Living building instead of her house, she knew exactly what was going on. The door of the suite opened and there sat my parents' furniture, bed, clothing, and the custom drapes. Mom was beyond angry! Dad wept and hugged me in appreciation. Taking me aside, he admitted it was the right move, but accepting everything was a difficult proposition.

Driving up to Mom & Dad's house was always beautiful; ninety minutes on a peninsula highway, followed by a twenty minute ferry ride and another twenty-five minutes to the door. Of course, that was based on "good day", encountering zero traffic. Immediately following my parents' move into the Assisted Living, I repeated that sequence two to three times each week, until both of them displayed some sense of contentment.

Equally as important and on my agenda was taking measures to empty out and clean their newly vacated residence and ready it for resale. There are no words to accurately describe the amount of paraphernalia the two of them had accumulated. Living abroad and with Mom being the consummate "hostess with the mostest", one can only imagine the amount of dishes and linens that were acquired, and then left behind. I arranged for the higher ticket items to be picked up by an auction house; my generous girlfriends bought several things; some pieces sold through advertisements; and I donated the remainder to a local parish. What I came away with following the experience: "Out of future consideration for those who may be left to liquidate your belongings, please downsize!"

Upon returning home after the final load was picked up, I received a cryptic phone call from a Parish volunteer who had been at the house earlier that day and charged with emptying Mom's linen closet. Acting very mysteriously, the woman claimed she had something important to speak with me about, but would only do so in person. As expected, I traipsed back up in the morning to meet with her. When I arrived, she jumped out of her car and handed me an envelope containing six thousand dollars in cash. It appears that for some time, my mom had been hiding one hundred dollar bills inside of a bag of cotton balls. While sorting through our donated items, this honorable soul found the money and immediately contacted me; bless her heart.

Jim died a few months after the move into the facility, which was a mere three days shy of their thirtieth anniversary. Throughout the funeral service, Mom kept asking me where Dad was, and I would respond that he was in Heaven. She would lower her head and say, "Oh, that's right." Later that evening, the family gathered for dinner at a local restaurant, and as we got up to leave, Mom turned around and said, "Where's Poppa? We can't leave without him." Grabbing her hand, I gently reminded her once again and it was heart-wrenching. That pair was truly meant to be together. They were good for each other and very much in love. My belief will always be that Dad was holding on for her. Now that she was safe and cared for, he could let go.

Following Jim's passing, my trips to see Mom once again became frequent. The disease was progressing and I began receiving a surplus of calls concerning her behavioral changes. Without fail, I'd drive back up to investigate. Most of the occurrences made me laugh. For instance, there was the time when she decided not to wear a bra, and instead, "MacGyver" fashioned her own by placing Band Aids over her nipples. JoAnn was so proud of her ingenuity that she raced to share it with everyone at the nurse's station. Lifting up her top, she addressed the staff with an enthusiastic, "What do you think of these?" Hilarious as that was to me, I was laughing alone. Because my mom wasn't residing in an Alzheimer's designated facility, events such as this soon developed into a series of complications.

RESUMING

Stress from the loss of her husband accelerated the progression tremendously. My mother wasn't answering her phone, nor showing up for meals. Convinced she was falling into a depression, I made my way up to administer a "pep talk". I gave her a lecture that could only have rivaled one of her own. Did I mention "tough love sucks?" Thankfully, it is also effective. She picked herself up and once again, joined the land of the living.

Always the social butterfly, JoAnn began to attend every possible event that was offered. In fact, trying to reach her by phone was almost impossible because she was never in her room. Actually, that pleased me. Once each week, the residents were offered various excursions on the Activity bus and you could bet, she didn't miss a trip. She didn't miss a meal either! Have you ever experienced mealtime at an Assisted Living facility? I liken it to renting a horse at the beach. Usually they are

charged out by the hour and you are able to select the level of horse most closely suited to your
skill level. Once sixty minutes have passed, with no
prodding, the horse does an about face and trans-
forms into Spectacular Bid, making his way back
to the starting line. I have just described the 5:00
p.m. mealtime in my mom's AL. The hallway became a sea of walkers, wheelchairs, and each cane-
clad resident metamorphosed into Carl Lewis.
Taking in the entire experience of feeding time
always made me smile. Every day this drill was repeated for fear they would miss their meal or lose
their spot, in spite of the fact that everyone had
pre-assigned tables.

It was wonderful to see Mom participating in so
many things and smiling again. The color had finally returned to her cheeks and her weight had
risen a bit. Due to exercise being limited in her
Assisted Living facility, she became inventive; walking the halls of the building several times each
day, taking the stairs from floor-to-floor. "I'm
walking around inside because I know I'm not allowed to go out alone", was her explanation to me.
Outwardly, aside from the forgetfulness, it wasn't
really apparent that she had Alzheimer's disease,
but the subtle behavioral changes spoke volumes
to me.

A prime example: Residents moving into the AL
were issued their apartment keys on a keychain

resembling an old-style phone cord. This would enable them to put it on like a bracelet and slide it up around their arm, ensuring that it was in a safe place and would not get lost. In its inception, this was a valid idea, but certainly not a great solution for everyone. Several times each week, Mom could not locate her key and would become frantic. The staff would patiently escort her back to the room, unlock her door and conduct a brief search. Completely frustrated and with no key in sight, JoAnn would make the decision to call it a night, asking the caregivers to leave. But, as soon as the staff had gone, she would hit my number on the speed dial to report what had transpired. Because this happened so often, I had my script down. Every time, I ran through the same battery of questions; where were you last? Did you put it down somewhere? Was it in your possession when you left the room? In an effort to solve the mystery, I'd ask her to place her hand at the top of her shoulder and run it down each arm. Miraculously her key would reappear, strapped to her upper arm. Feeling ridiculous, she would toss out an expletive and we'd both laugh; yes, each and every time.

W-T-F

The Alzheimer's secured residence was located directly across the parking lot from the Assisted Living building. Endeavoring to create a sense of community, the caregivers would often arrange combined social events. My mom attended all of them and on numerous occasions was so busy socializing, she'd miss the call to head back to the other building. After dark, she would appear at the door like a puppy, waiting for security to let her into the main lobby. Incidences such as this made me very uneasy, but in most respects she still wasn't ready for "maximum lock-up"; at least, not from my perspective.

The fun continued when a new female resident was temporarily moved into the Assisted Living. Her short stay in my mom's building met with many challenges, specifically social. She really didn't smile or speak, and her lack of expression was misinterpreted as unfriendliness. In actuality, the poor thing was expressing fear and confusion. Mom took to her, for whatever reason, and they became friends. Early one afternoon, during another combined social event, JoAnn decided that a trip to the beach was in order. Note that the AL residence was situated about three miles from Puget Sound and had a peek-a-boo view of the water. So, based on the judgment of this adventurous duo, if they could see it from the deck, it must be close. To this day, I have no idea how they were able to slip out, but approximately two hours later, the ladies showed up at a local Burger King, neither with an inkling of where her home was located. It wasn't long, after a short game of Twenty Questions, that a Good Samaritan solved the puzzle and drove them back.

As new behaviors presented themselves, the phone calls to me increased in number. Endeavoring to keep my eye on the ball and observe JoAnn in person, I made the journey up once each month, to take her out for a meal and shopping. She really looked forward to our dates, as did I. It may not sound that exciting, but it never mattered what we did, as long as we were together. Door-to-door the trip took roughly 2¾ hours, so I would depart at 6:00 a.m. and return home around 8:30 p.m. The short-term memory loss was becoming increasingly pronounced, so as back-up, I would always schedule two reminder calls en route. The first was made while aboard the ferry and the second, from seven minutes out. One time, adhering to my ritual, I arrived only to discover that a mere three minutes after we had spoken, the social butterfly had happily boarded the facility's Activity bus and was to be gone for the next several hours. I did the only thing I could do - laugh and begin the sojourn home.

A similar event took place one Easter. Our family had planned to take her out to brunch, but upon our arrival, we found her seated and participating in the Assisted Living's holiday luncheon, sipping a glass of champagne. Even funnier was the fact that this was the second seating; she had already eaten, yet had no memory of being at the first meal, so was settling in for round two. Although our visit had been planned for a month, we were greeted with a warm "Well for Heaven's sake! What are you doing here?"

Each passing month continued to cultivate new challenges and questions, as to whether or not the Assisted Living was still the right fit. Mom's needs had definitely increased, yet she remained happy, oblivious and reasonably self-sufficient.

THE LITTLE BITCHES
THAT CLEAN

Coming from a household where laughter was our pharmaceutical of choice, I quickly began to discover the humorous side of certain behaviors. When a small child does something that makes no sense at all, we find it amusing, taking delight in the moment. Not unlike that innocent being is an individual afflicted with Alzheimer's. Their actions are perfectly in-line to them, but not always to us. Isn't it more constructive to board their fantasy flight and truly enjoy them while we have the opportunity?

Somewhere between the second and third stages, Mom began exhibiting a great deal of paranoia. Hiding items of importance to her became the norm. Cosmetics, scarves, jewelry, foundations; you name it, she tucked it away. Replenishing her supplies proved fruitless, as they too went missing. Convinced that it must be the cleaning crew, she labeled them as "the little bitches that clean." Not wanting to dismiss Mom's concerns, nor embarrass her, I offered to conduct ongoing investigations. Each time I would proceed directly over to the top dresser drawer, reach in beneath the same exact pile of scarves, and voila! I'd uncover a treasure trove of missing items. Gently, I'd point out that she may have taken the lead on the concealment, but she forever stuck to her theory.

Toilet tissue, paper towel and laundry soap were not supplied, so we would stop at Costco on our way to visit her and stock up. We always made certain she had enough to last her for a couple of weeks. Well, apparently the "bitches" were at it again, because a few of those items disappeared as well. The missing toilet paper presented an even greater challenge to the facility, as it prompted Mom to alternatively begin using paper towels. Needless to say, her commode was deemed "Out-of-Order" around forty percent of the time, and the building maintenance crew was being summoned like clockwork. Again donning my detective's persona, I set out to locate the hidden loot, rifling through the cupboards and closets. At last, success! Inside her bedroom closet, fifteen rolls of much needed toilet tissue were discovered, alongside the laundry detergent and her missing pillows.

The paradoxical behaviors continued to thrive. A specific instance I found to be truly ironic, was when Mom decided to hide her apartment key in a "safer" location. Yes, the same one that was usually strapped around her upper arm and continually MIA. Since keeping it on her person didn't seem to be working out very well, she made the decision to place it in an undisclosed location; this time, outside of her door.

On one of our late October jaunts to the drugstore, she purchased a stuffed pumpkin-head doll. It had the body of a toddler, an oversized pumpkin-head, and around its arm hung a tiny pumpkin-shaped candy basket. Contrived of cloth, wire, and polyester stuffing, standing approximately 3 ½ ft. tall, it assumed the roles of watchman, welcoming committee, and keeper of the key. In plain sight she would place the key to her room inside of the pumpkin-head's trick or treat basket. The same woman who was convinced the housekeepers were stealing, thought she was hiding her key in a locale that surely no one would think to look. She may have been correct, as no one, including JoAnn, could find it! Her thought process was admirable, but her methods confused. And yes, the speed dial began getting a workout, yet again.

As the winter settled in, we wanted to make her little apartment even cozier. My brother brought her a flat screen television and set it up in the bedroom. He ordered cable and additional movie channels for her, envisioning that she would crawl into her bed each evening and drift off to either Frank Sinatra or Montgomery Clift. Best laid plans . . . Despite being profoundly appreciative, she could not figure out how to operate the new controls. That was understandable, as navigating around those things can get confusing for any-one. I made a color-coded key for her with step-by-step instructions and placed it on her table for easy access. Within a week, the reference guide I had made for her went missing (most likely the "bitches") and my phone began ringing off the hook on a regular schedule. Thank God I have a photographic memory, because I was able to walk her through the sequence night after night. That is, until she began misplacing the remote controls.

Relaying Mom's frustration to my brother, he de-cided to purchase two tiny alarms for her and at-tach them to the remotes. Each alarm consisted of a key fab & ringer counterpart. Using a signifi-cant amount of duct tape, he strapped the ringer to each remote control and taped the fab to her dresser. Should one of the remotes vanish, she could press a button on the ringer component and a little alarm would sound on the TV control.

Sounds simple, but it was very confusing to Mom. Her calls would continue to come at their usu-al time; however, now I would be charged with locating her TV controls via the telephone. The directions were always the same: she was asked to walk over to her dresser and press one of the two key fab buttons, simultaneously holding the phone in the air. Mom would comply and I could hear the faint sound of an alarm going off in the other room. The phone was a cordless, so she would put down the handset and go into the living room to look. That's when I thought we were good-to-go, and that's when we ran into a wall. I'd hear "Oh, for God's sake" and a giggle. Now she'd lost the handset. Envision me calling out at the top of my lungs countless times through the receiver, "Mom, I'm here," until finally, we were back on the line. Her next words to me would be, "When did I become such a numb-nuts?" We'd laugh together, while repeating the entire process. Eventually, we removed the television from the bedroom.

AND YOU ARE?

Individuals in the early stages of Alzheimer's seem to be surprisingly aware of the ongoing struggle with their memories. My observation has been that in an effort to mask their lack of recall and the embarrassment that accompanies it, each cultivates a little bag of tricks. These tools present themselves in a variety of forms: a laugh in lieu of a response; acquiescing to alternate points of view, merely to avoid a possible challenge; crafting extremely convincing tales on the fly; and in my mother's case, false recognition. This "acknowledgement" manifested itself in the form of kissing and hugging total strangers, as though they were long lost friends. Let me preface this by stating that because JoAnn was always a highly demonstrative individual, this behavior was not out of the ordinary. She did, however, continue to surprise us with the number of new occurrences, coupled with her increasing lack of lingual inhibition.

Not unlike many Alzheimer's sufferers, there did come a point when Mom began to think that everyone looked familiar. Irrespective of where we were, she would walk directly over to someone and say, "Oh, honey, it is so great to see you. Do you remember me? I'm JoAnn." Usually, we'd slip behind her, motioning our arms back and forth, simultaneously mouthing an apology. It was amazing to me how generous some individuals could be. The moment they ascertained what was happening, they began to play along, solely out of graciousness. And to be clear, we were never ashamed of her, merely protective.

One afternoon, I had driven Mom over to a local drugstore to browse. My back had been turned for approximately twenty seconds, when I heard her speaking with someone. Quickly rounding the corner, there stood my 5'4"mother, in front of a 6'4" African American gentleman, with her fingers entwined in his two-inch cornrows. Initially he wasn't smiling, perhaps because he was startled. However, soon after, he broke into a wide grin when he recognized that she was genuinely interested in the construction process behind his hairdo. "You look just darling," is all she kept stating. "I'd like to do that to my hair." Yes, my tiny mother with her blonde, bulletproof "mom" wig and bright smile sporting cornrows? That would truly be something to behold! Silently expressing my amends, I swiftly escorted her away to cosmetics department and distracted her with the makeup.

Advancing into Stage Three, JoAnn had now completely lost her verbal filter. Not that she owned a strong one prior to this, but "wow!" Albeit always outspoken and a bit of a stinker, she did at one time possess a modicum of self-control. Well, that had vanished completely! The majority of the time, her remarks were highly amusing, but not always. For instance, one time when my brother went up for a visit, he and Mom stopped by her bank branch to handle some business before lunch. While waiting to be helped, she spied a woman in line ahead of them that she swore was a friend. My mother was off like a shot to speak to the gal, and cupping the woman's face in her hands, she remarked on cue, "How are you, honey? It's been so long. Remember me? I'm JoAnn. Boy, have you ever gotten fat." My brother was rendered speechless, and the arm-waving commenced. Fortunately, the woman was very understanding. When the story was relayed to me, I laughed and offered up a healthy serving of "Welcome to my world." Similar to a toddler verbally parroting an inappropriate phrase, Alzheimer's disease transports the individual back to that point of innocence, where unsuitable statements necessitate nothing more than instant forgiveness.

Another attribute in this particular stage, at least through my observation, was the "pride in owner-ship" that Mom began exhibiting. Apparently un-beknownst to the family, by her account she was now the proud owner of the Assisted Living facility in which she resided. JoAnn continually reassured us that she was being well attended to, and if at any point the staff dropped the ball, they would be let go. Well, that certainly made me feel better. In fact, it seemed that she had secretly invested in a number of properties in the region, including an apartment building and the local diner that she used to frequent. Obviously, I'm being facetious. During the progression of this disease, some af-flicted individuals will arrive at a juncture where they come to believe that they're holding the deed to everything. I can't be certain, but it seems plau-sible that feeling completely in charge of their cur-rent surroundings is a way of compensating for the underlying sense of losing control.

Not to be forgotten was the "Love is in the Air" page of the script. An abundance of male suitors, were relentlessly pursuing Mom – at least, that's what she reported to me. Always a big fan of the opposite gender, my mother suddenly sparked an interest in a few of the male residents, and they in her. This was worrisome for a split second, until I saw them for myself. Each admirer maintained his own mobility aid; one used a walker, another had a wheelchair and the third, my mom's favorite, drove around on an electric scooter. I'm certain buzzing around the halls on his ride, was the attraction. As expected, it didn't take long before JoAnn announced that she held the title for that shiny beast parked at the end of the hall.

What became blatantly clear was that in this particular stage of the Alzheimer's progression, many individuals once again launched into their sexual prime. It isn't that Mom was actually doing anything about it, but I did start receiving feedback from the caregivers about a couple of unexplained and prolonged absences during the late afternoon. When questioned about where she went when she disappeared, JoAnn would smile and avoid any direct eye contact. Reading between the lines, she obviously had no memory of those supposed trysts, but thoroughly enjoyed the attention and mystery.

Personally, I have been witness to several hand-holding sessions and on a couple of occasions, instances where she flat-out planted a big smooch on a male resident, who clearly was flirting with her. Since none of these behaviors was malicious, or tawdry, no action was required. Occurrences such as these only become an issue when there is a lack of understanding about the disease. Our loved ones are in their home and among others in the same mental space. They are living, breathing creatures with the same physiological needs as they have always had. Actually, they are responding to each other in a "normal" manner. The only thought I ever had was "You go, Mom."

JoAnn's world became such a wonderland - magical, innocent, pure, and safe (sans the "little bitches"). Each and every visit would exhibit something new. A simple walk down a hallway would develop into a lengthy story-telling session with Mom pointing out various characters in a random wall hanging and providing the history behind the art, as it related to her childhood. The cat in the photo became her cat and the sailboat, her grandfather's. Some of the tales were fashioned from events that actually did take place. For example, the story would begin with an event that took place in 1982 and then an account from 1975 would be added. Voila, the birth of yet another brand new experience. Both, I had been present for; just not in the manner in which they were introduced. JoAnn was always a "colorful" raconteur, but Alzheimer's had bumped her into another league.

Perhaps the most difficult incident to-date transpired during this stage. I had planned to take Mom to lunch one day at a nearby restaurant, only to have her look at me without recognition, walk right past me, and head out of the door. Just when I thought I had it all under control, here was a cold reminder that I was human and "this was happening." I had been quite confident that my feelings were in check, but hadn't anticipated the failure of recognition this soon.

PART I: IN SEARCH OF

When JoAnn was initially diagnosed, she was the resident of a small town and under the care of the local family doctor. Most of Mom's friends in the area went to the same clinic and they all seemed to trust him. That's all well and fine, but he was not a specialist in either Geriatrics or Alzheimer's, so I made a point of setting up her next appointment and accompanying her to his office. My reasons were three-fold: First, I wanted to introduce myself; second, I wished to discuss her treatment regimen with him; third, I needed to look him directly in the eye and provide him with a head's up: Should I ever arrive at my mother's residence and find that she was glazed over due to a prescription, he could be sure to expect a visit from me. Perhaps it was because I had watched too many movies where patients were "snowed", or over-medicated. Maybe it was a direct result of discovering that, during a prior visit, he prescribed two Alzheimer's medications at the same time. Whatever the reason, I felt it was my duty to make certain that the pharmaceutical Band-Aid was being administered properly.

My next visit up to see Mom became the straw that broke the camel's back, so to speak. Walking in to fetch her from the lobby of her building per the usual routine, it became apparent that something was off. If you have ever owned a cat, you understand that during play and immediately before they pounce, their eyes dilate, turning black and glassy. That is exactly how her eyes looked. Now, combine that with the foam appearing in the corners of her mouth and her slurred speech, you have the perfect storm, pharmaceutically speaking, and true to my word, I set forth to pay the doctor the visit I'd promised him.

Pulling off to the side of the road to get a good look at her, I was disgusted. She could barely articulate, and her speech was not only slurred, it was delivered in slow motion. It killed me to see this otherwise smiley, chatty, extremely happy woman, reduced to a zombie. Throughout the course of the day, the medication began to wear off and the fog started to lift. There's no way to express how upset I was, but reacting at that exact moment would not have been constructive. I'm a firm believer in allowing one's self an adequate amount of time to cool off and regain perspective before a necessary confrontation. That morning was no exception.

After spending the better part of the day with Mom, I dropped her off at her residence and headed straight to her doctor's office. Arriving without an appointment, as expected, they were less than pleased to see me. All right, maybe that wasn't the only reason. The contentious tone of my voice made it quite clear that I was less than enamored with the services JoAnn had received and had no intention of leaving without a dialog with her doctor. They expeditiously ushered me into an exam room to remove me from within earshot of the patients in the Waiting area. Much to my disappointment, in walked the doctor's associate, as the individual I came to see was suddenly unavailable. With no hesitation, my planned statement was expressed and I exited with Mom's medical records in-hand.

OK, it sounds like I was being an overprotective, intolerant bitch. My abruptness may be interpreted as such; but I'm a straight-shooter. What no one can ever accuse me of is neglecting, ignoring, or failing in my role as my mother's advocate, friend and loving daughter. My mission to find her a new physician immediately commenced. Specific areas I searched in were Geriatrics, Gastroenterology and Dementia/Alzheimer's. In no time at all, Mom had a new doctor, who fortunately specialized in all three.

JoAnn's first appointment was challenging, to say the least. As she was a new patient, they wanted to conduct a series of tests to properly diagnose her. At this point, my only thought was, *Are they serious? She has already been through "those" tests, but I suppose we're here now.* Garnering every last ounce of my patience, I sat quietly by Mom's side and held her hand as the testing began. The first task assigned to her was to repeat from memory five different words that the medical assistant had recited for her, three minutes prior. Looking to me for help was common, but I assured her she could do this on her own. Giggling nervously, she could only remember one of them. To be completely honest, I could only come up with four. That made her laugh and eased some of the embarrassment. Next, they asked her a slew of questions for which she had only a handful of answers, and again, I wasn't allowed to help.

Finally, the nurse administered the Clox test; an assessment designed to screen for cognitive impairment. Individuals are asked to draw the face of a clock inside of a large circle on the back of a form, with the hands displaying the time of 1:45 p.m. Additional instruction or prompting is not allowed. What a heart-wrenching exercise to observe. How could something so profoundly simple, be such a struggle? In the end, JoAnn drew an incredibly detailed smiley face, complete with eyelashes, which was always her signature drawing. Phoning my brother with a recounting of the examination, all I had to do was mention a "smiley face" and he asked me if she drew eyelashes. Everything about that visit was simultaneously sad and dear.

Our sessions with the doctor would continue to take place approximately every thirty to forty days. JoAnn underwent the same testing ritual each visit. Eventually, the day arrived when it became flagrantly clear to me, she'd had enough. How many smiley faces did she have to draw? By some miracle did they expect her to improve? She was still in the early stages and fairly cognizant of everything. Avoiding further humiliation for her, I put an end to the testing.

Finding the 'perfect fit' doctor-wise wasn't smooth sailing. Just as you would hope to feel some type of connection with your own physician, I wanted that for Mom. Initially, the doctor that we chose was brilliant. Also blatantly obvious was that he knew a lot about electronics. Yes, that fact was crystal clear because his laptop, desktop and cell phone were the only things he looked at during the appointment. Not once did he engage with either of us when speaking, in fact, I'm not certain I would recognize him on the street, unless, of course, he had his back to me. His Bluetooth was perched over his left ear and I recall Mom saying, "Excuse me, Sir, what is that little thing in your ear?" Without flinching (or turning around), he stated that it was his phone. She looked at me and shrugged her shoulders, as she'd never seen a Bluetooth device before.

Her next comment was priceless: "Sir, I'm sorry I'm such an idiot," and that apparently was the golden ticket. He stopped typing, finally spinning his chair around to make his first eye contact of the appointment with Mom. In response he assured her that she was not an idiot, recognizing that his actions had suggested otherwise. Yes, JoAnn was still aware – aware of exactly what she was doing, which delighted me. She was a master at delivering the covert "fuck you," artfully concealed beneath her childlike gaze and beautiful smile.

We never saw that doctor again, but tried seeing one of his associates for at least a few more visits. Eventually, I found the right fit in a female physician close to my home. She was knowledgeable, as well as kind, and treated my mother with respect. In fact, during JoAnn's first appointment, as the doctor placed the stethoscope on her back, Mom said, "Oooh, can you scratch?" Without hesitation, the lovely doctor smiled and began doing just that. She continued with her exam and made my mom feel very comfortable. It's so important to remember that simply because an individual has developed Alzheimer's it does not mean he or she is devoid of feelings, nor should they be treated with any less regard than you or I.

PART II: IN SEARCH OF

Simultaneously, when I was searching for my mom's physician, the quest to locate a new living situation ensued. Let me just state that the process is an eye-opener. Internet research was first on the agenda, enabling me to devise a game plan. However, there were a number of factors that needed to be taken into consideration when looking for the appropriate residence: The stage of AD Mom was in; Were there other residents at that same level; What did the daily agenda consist of i.e., spiritual services, activities schedule, field trips, mental stimulation, as well as physical exercise; meal plan; cleanliness of facility; insurance programs accepted (if any); Medicaid-eligible facility, or private; staff-to-resident ratio. Those elements are highly important, but the number one benchmark in my opinion, had everything to do with the employees. In dealing with this type of disease, a caregiver has to "get it." A rare individual possessing an enormous amount of compassion and patience is essential to working within this environment. Your loved one deserves nothing less than to be treated with respect and enabled to prevail with their dignity intact. Is that too tall of an order? No, I don't believe so. None of these loving souls adopted this existence; it chose them.

Retirement facilities often offer three separate levels of care: Independent Living, Memory Care and Assisted. Generally, a Nurse's station is located inside of the main building, where daily medicines are dispensed and administered. Each property sports an Activity area and Formal Dining room and a few are equipped with a Social Lounge, Beauty Salon and Exercise room. A base fee is charged for the apartment and a bevy of add-on options are available. The final price-tag depends entirely on the type of care one is seeking and the amount of assistance they require, but be well-prepared for sticker-shock! Bells and whistles aside, the selection process requires an enormous leap of faith on your part, as first impressions aren't always accurate. Trust me!!

Following my research, a list of potential facilities that I wished to tour was drafted. None presented that well online, but they all offered a combination of comforts I knew would please Mom. Setting up appointments with each, the touring commenced. Outside of the confirmation that Mom did indeed have Alzheimer's, entering these facilities was the second most disturbing period for me. My primary concern was figuring out what type of residence she needed. Could she live on her own, or should Mom be behind secured doors? In my heart, I was convinced she wasn't there yet, but I kept an open mind. While JoAnn needed some help, she was not quite ready for "lock-up", so the decision was made to stick with an Assisted Living facility, plus the addition of a few extra services.

RED FLAGS ABOUND

Driving up to Mom's newly selected residence, we got the sense that we were arriving at a six-star resort. The perfectly manicured grounds were lovely and adorned handsomely with statuary. The building by itself was beautiful, especially the interior. From the moment we approached the automatic sliding doors under the large covered entryway and stepped into the pristine lobby, everything spoke to luxury. Clearly the building had been professionally decorated. Floral arrangements were abundant, the furnishings high-end, wallpaper stunning, and the two dining rooms lavishly appointed. Included were all of the perks one could imagine, such as a study, computer room, indoor pool, whirlpool spa, hair salon, exercise area, soda fountain, putting green and gift shop; each conveniently located under one roof. It was an enormous structure divided into two sides; one for Independent Living residents and the other for those requiring an Assisted Living situation.

Yes, this was surely the right place for my mother, or so I was led to believe.

Moving day finally arrived and I was thrilled. Visiting my Mom would now constitute nothing more than a twelve minute drive, as opposed to the former 2¾ hour trek. I left my home at 6:00 in the morning to retrieve her on the island, and we arrived at her new living quarters later that afternoon. It is important to note that during the initial meeting with the administration team at the new residence, I had been extremely forthcoming about my mother's Alzheimer's. Sticking to protocol, they had also invited Mom in for a mandatory assessment.

Following that evaluation, we collectively decided that it would be best to move her into a room within close proximity to the Nurse's Station. Herein is where the downward spiral began. You see, they had sold themselves as a facility that was fully equipped to handle a candidate with Alzheimer's disease and we had no reason to question their qualifications. Despite asking all of the right questions (and believe me, I did), we were completely deceived. Basically, we tossed our hearts out onto the table, alongside the checkbook, and they pounced like a lion onto a piece of meat.

The first of many red flags presented itself when they told us (on moving day) that it was going to be a problem to place Mom into an apartment near the Nurse's Station; as previously discussed, because they had nothing available. And even if they did, it would be significantly more costly. With this type of facility, the monthly rate is exceedingly expensive and we were already dealing with that harsh reality. But we had made the commitment, so we accepted a beautiful little one bedroom apartment on the lower floor at the end of a hallway.

For an individual under ordinary circumstances this unit would have been perfect. The location was around the corner from the elevators, kitty-corner from the laundry room, and directly down the hallway from the door to the parking lot. Our immediate concerns were that Mom was being presented with a great deal of change all at once, and her memory was failing miserably. As familiarity is oxygen to an Alzheimer's candidate, how would she react to this change? She had been walking the same path to her room in her previous residence for the past couple of years and her short term memory was declining. I was so worried that she would not be able to retrain herself to head down from the main level in an elevator, instead of up to the second floor. Behind her glance was a scared little girl, and my heart simply ached.

We explored other available options that would address our concerns and provide the level of care my mother required. Every organization operates differently, but this particular facility sold extra caretaking in blocks, or packages. Depending on how much care was required, each block would cost approximately $300; we chose to pay for two. This would entitle us to having Mom escorted from her room to all activities and meals, and then returned safely. Medications would be administered daily, her hair coiffed once each week in the facility's salon, and every other day an attendant would stand by in her room while she showered, in the event of a fall. Yes, $600 additional each month for a little extra assistance, which, I soon discovered, she was not receiving.

My first inkling of this was when I encountered a horrible stench in her apartment upon on of my visits. Searching everywhere for the source, I finally came across a few pair of soiled undies hidden in the back corner of the walk-in closet. Unfortunately, any extra help we had been promised and were paying for was nonexistent. Mom had experienced a couple of "accidents" and lacked the rationale to deal with her dirty clothing, so she tucked it in the closet behind her shoes. The poor thing was in such a state of confusion after the recent move, she didn't know which end was up. That is specifically why we were forthright with the administration team from the onset. Mom needed help!

Regarding the escort to and from meals, we found that although we had paid the staff to fetch her, if she expressed any indication of not being prepared to go at that specific moment, she didn't eat. That was interesting, given that in the facility's brochure, they clearly stated that twenty four hour dining was available. Perhaps we misunderstood and they meant in and around the area, not in their dining room. In a period of less than three weeks, Mom had dropped approximately eighteen pounds. This may sound like a gross exaggeration, but I assure you, it is not.

As mentioned, the interior décor was gorgeous; each area was adorned perfectly within a consistent theme. That said, trying to distinguish one floor from the next became extremely challenging; each was an exact replica of the other. It was very easy for all of us to become disoriented, so I could only imagine how Mom must have felt, poor thing. Endeavoring to provide her with a point of reference, so she could locate her new room, I placed a pretty eucalyptus wreath on her door. This wreath held a special significance, because I had made it as a gift for her several years prior and decorated it with shells that we had collected together on a beach in Florida.

It marked her door, but more importantly, it provided a memory. In her previous building, we used it for the same purpose and quite successfully;

she always found her apartment. Now that she'd moved, there was a sense of comfort knowing that the wreath was back on her door. That, coupled with the additional assistance we were funding, would ensure that she could find her room and furnish her with a feeling of security.

Yeah, right. For the record, I arrived one day within the first week of her residency to find the wreath missing. The staff had been instructed to move it to the inside of her apartment, because it conflicted with the building's décor. The wreath itself was lovely, but even if it wasn't, that was disrespectful. A sinking feeling came over me. Is this what the administration meant by "We are equipped to handle Alzheimer's?" Needless to say, the family was disappointed.

Now that I was closer in proximity, a short visit each day through the adjustment period was not out of the question. Logically, I knew that she was OK, but just the idea that she might be afraid made me sad. At a minimum, if she saw my face, a friendly one, the degree of loneliness perhaps would dissipate. Still learning to navigate the corridors, each mirroring the next, she would venture out for her daily exercise, walking the halls and climbing each stairway. Mom had been including this activity in her daily routine for quite some time, as previously mentioned, because I suggested she refrain from going outdoors by herself. For some unknown reason that particular advice stuck and I was thankful, however, the staff would soon form a different opinion.

Mom seemed to be adequately settling in to her new accommodations, however if you asked her, she would always respond that she was ready to go home. Getting her head around the simple fact that she was already there, simply wasn't happening. Hindsight tells me that if she had truly been happy, even in spite of the memory issues, the adjustment would have been less difficult.

The door to the parking lot sat at the opposite end of JoAnn's hallway. This is the exact same door that I always used when picking her up to go out. Week two, following her move-in date, she woke up in the middle of the night, highly confused; not uncommon with Alzheimer's, especially when familiarity has been compromised. She proceeded to get out of bed, dress herself, don the wig, put on lipstick, and head over to the door to wait for me. Under the impression I was on the way at 2:30 a.m., no less, my mother exited the building to make sure I wasn't waiting for her around the corner. When she didn't find me, Mom headed back to the door, only to find it locked. Now, imagine yourself alone, in an unfamiliar place, in the dark. Under normal circumstances that may be a bit daunting, but toss Alzheimer's into the mix. She was frightened, but had the wherewithal to walk around this large building to the front entrance, in an effort to regain access. It was also locked, but she persisted in knocking on the glass doors until a security guard eventually let her back into the facility.

Immediately after, the administrative staff wasted no time at all in documenting this incident and placing it in JoAnn's file. They labeled her a "flight risk" and stated that she tried to "flee" from the building. What's even more alarming to me is that they were not even the slightest bit interested in listening to an explanation. According to my mother, she felt like an idiot.

JoAnn's previous dwelling was quite a bit smaller and easier to maneuver through. But, she now was starting to accept that this new building was her home. Traveling around the corridors was like moving throughout her house and seemed perfectly logical. Mom was known for strolling around in one of her many ornate caftans, in full make-up and wearing her "not a hair out of place" wig. Smelling of perfume and soap, every nail was perfectly painted, lipstick in place, and her body iced with just the right amount of jewelry. Visually, she was a beautiful woman and inside, even more so.

Well, Mom's daily "activity" did not bode well with the management, and I began getting pummeled with phone calls saying, "Your mom did this" or

"Your mom did that." I hadn't seen anything in the brochure that stated, "Walking the hallways is prohibited." Okay, so there was an instance in which she tried to enter another room that, coincidentally, happened to be in the exact location of her apartment in the former locale. Three questions sprang to mind: 1) Were we not upfront about our concerns & paying extra? 2) Where did you say the wreath went? 3) You did say you had the professional chops to deal with Alzheimer's, correct? Bottom line was that my mother would rather walk around exploring and visiting with people than sit in a chair and toss a beach ball back and forth. Shame on her! This did not go over well with the staff, as they were now obligated to pay attention.

Grievances kept pouring in about Mom and running out of subjects to complain about, it now fell to her choice of apparel. The administrators felt that it was highly inappropriate for her to walk around in a caftan. I'm not delusional, she really did look beautiful and wasn't this her home? The particular garments in question were purchased for entertaining, similar to the cocktail pant back in the day and were very ornate. Unfortunately, this organization had a reputation to uphold, and Mom was putting a crimp in the chain. Bandera roja!

Still trying to establish my own footing with this disease called Alzheimer's and the baggage that accompanied it, I was becoming extremely annoyed with the surplus of grievances heading my direction. Certain staff members continually berating my mom, coupled with the fact that we were paying in excess of $5500 each month and nothing was going as smoothly as we'd been promised, really infuriated me. As one does, I decidedly became a fixture during her transition period to afford myself a birds-eye view of what was really occurring. In my mind I was being proactive and in theirs, a giant pain in the ass.

BREAKING MOM

Alzheimer's disease has a nasty way of progressing rapidly, then pulling back. Contrary to how it might appear from one day to the next, our loved ones are not going to get better. Continually adapting falls onto the caregiver. Unfortunately, the stress of the past year in combination with the shoddy treatment Mom was receiving exacerbated her condition and her outlook became bleak. At least the holidays were approaching, which would supply some much needed excitement.

Thanksgiving Day arrived and I headed over to JoAnn's early in the morning to get her moving. We had made reservations for the family to enjoy brunch together and I wanted to ensure Mom was ready on time. History had taught me that she always moved like a turtle, but that was fine and I had no intention of rushing her. Once her outfit of the day was selected and she was out of the shower, I headed straight back to my home to ready myself for the festivities. I returned to her apartment approximately forty minutes later, only to discover that she was nowhere to be found. The entire family began searching the building in the obvious places, as well as stairwells, common areas and lastly, the dining room. There she sat in all of her glory, surrounded by a table full of someone else's relatives, with a huge crab leg protruding from her mouth. "Well, for heaven's sake. What are you doing here? I didn't know you were coming."

Yes, that was her greeting. The all too familiar, sweet welcome with no recollection of the time we had spent together earlier that morning, or that we were taking her to brunch. Neither my husband, nor I would dream of making Mom feel bad, so we proceeded to pull up two chairs, introduced ourselves to her "new friends" and visited with her while she ate. Repeatedly throughout the brunch, she would ask us to explain why we were not breaking bread with her on a holiday. Happy Thanksgiving!

The following day was fairly uneventful, until midday when the phone rang. It was Nurse Ratchet (the RN in charge from Mom's residence) and she appeared to be highly agitated. I asked her to slow down her speech and start at the beginning. Listening intently to her version of what happened convinced me that I needed to get over there, as soon as possible. Knowing my mother better than anyone and understanding Alzheimer's and its inherent behaviors, there was a larger concern here that had little to do with JoAnn. Again, I wasn't wearing blinders, but enough was enough!

Entering my mom's apartment, I found her in her bed, blinds drawn, weeping uncontrollably. Anyone who has known JoAnn, would affirm that this was completely out of character. Something horrible had to have transpired to generate this volume of degradation. This beautiful, loving, and kind soul lay before me, utterly broken.

Prior to continuing, I feel it is very important to preface what I am about to share by pointing out that back in her forties, Mom had been diagnosed with colorectal cancer and had to have a large portion of her small colon removed. Whenever this type of procedure is performed, you are forced to adapt to physical changes. Enjoying a nice meal now meant light on the spice, easy on the dairy, and in close proximity to a washroom. Because we were too naïve at the time to understand the enormity of the situation, we teased her relentlessly. I've lost track of how many close calls she endured, in addition to "accidents," but there were many.

For instance, I recall one October taking her to a drugstore after lunch to pick up some goodies. A scarecrow on a stick caught my mother's eye, and, for whatever reason, she wanted me to buy it for her. Like a child with a new toy, Mom proudly marched her new hobgoblin around the store, up and down the aisles, as though she were leading a line of Olympic athletes into the stadium. Wherever you stood in the store, you could see that scarecrow held high, peeking his nose above the merchandise . . . and then it was gone. Racing over to the aisle she last occupied, I found her new treasure, flat on its side. On the floor I spied a faint trail of little drips leading back towards the pharmacy, then into the restroom. Yes, without warning, her lunch had run right through and the moment Mom recognized what was taking place, she ran. How humiliating to repeatedly have this happen, and all due to the hand you were dealt. The most amazing thing of all is that she never complained about having cancer, or the surgery. Instead, she counted her blessings and was thankful to be alive. I felt this was a viable side note to share, in order for you to fully appreciate what really took place the November day that "Broke" my mom.

The day after Thanksgiving, JoAnn headed out for her morning jaunt around the building. She had only been living there a few weeks and was still terribly confused when it came to the location of her room. As mentioned, the wreath was gone and everything looked exactly the same, but nonetheless Mom confidently traveled up and down the corridors, from one side of the facility to the next, and suddenly, she felt it; that all too familiar warm wave in her stomach, emerging with no forewarning. At this point in her walk, unbeknownst to her, she was in the Retirement Living side of the building and had no idea where the bathrooms were located. The residence is massive and there was no one around to ask, so she hurriedly pressed on down the hallway, her only mission finding the toilet. Regrettably, she didn't make it and found herself not only covered in waste, but mortified. Of course, had Mom been able to travel a mere fifteen additional yards down the hall, she would have found the lavatory.

In that moment, my mother wanted to run and hide, but being the woman she is, remarkably had the presence of mind to forge on until finally locating the washroom. Safely in a stall, she proceeded to remove her soiled slacks and underwear, and clean herself up. The contaminated clothing was such a mess, there was no point in putting it back on. Fortunately, she was a huge fan of longer tops, and in her thinking, pulling the sweater down to cover her bum area would at least suffice until she was able to locate the stairwell, which eventually she did. Note that Alzheimer's disease does not foster a rational thought process.

Temporarily out of sight, she made her way down the stairs at lightning speed, not really knowing where they would lead. The descent continued until there were no more stairs, and crossing her fingers this was the correct floor, she exited into the corridor. In tears, she breezed by an open door, which just so happened to be Nurse Ratchet's office. Mom heard her name and a loud, condescending, "What the hell do you think you're doing?" Weeping hysterically, which as I told you, was totally out of character for Mom, she attempted to offer an explanation, but the nurse wouldn't listen. Instead of comforting her, the unfeeling bitch scolded and belittled JoAnn. In fact, that nasty, insensitive woman reprimanded Mom all the way back to her apartment. And that was where she remained for the next few days; alone in her dark space, sobbing and completely shattered. It was also the very first time I had ever heard Mom say "I want to die."

Customary in nursing homes and senior living facilities is the documentation of out-of-the-ordinary incidents, which is then placed into the involved resident's chart. Now that you understand the circumstances, this is how the report was communicated: "Resident was found running around the building with no clothing on, defecating in the hallway." Are you kidding me? Nothing in the way of an explanation was attached. Of course, we know the truth, so why does it matter what is chronicled in your loved one's chart? Well, to begin, there's that little thing called "dignity," which, in my mother's case, the nurse took no steps to preserve. Additionally, should the day arrive when any decision is made to move Mom into a different facility, the documented "high maintenance" aspect may result in her being turned away.

Essentially, this particular individual made no effort to alleviate Mom's embarrassment, nor console her. What she did accomplish was breaking JoAnn. Furthermore, she booted her out of the residence. That's correct. My mother had been there for just under four weeks and they wanted to wash their hands of her. I was summoned to the facility's office and informed that she was no longer welcome and was given less than a week to get her out. Weren't these the exact same people who readily accepted our money and assured us that they were equipped to handle Alzheimer's? Difficult to imagine someone being this cold-hearted, but I assure you, my memory of that conversation is crystal clear.

Take a moment to imagine yourself in my mom's place, with your healthy, rational mind, facing a similar situation. On a daily basis, you are already enduring an abundance of snippy attitudes, demeaning glares, and disrespect, when an embarrassing mishap takes place. Despite the fact that your chart clearly outlines your pre-existing conditions, including your occasional untimely bowel movements, the staff elects to respond in the form of verbal attacks, making you feel worse than you already do, rather than being supportive, or re-spectful. Personally, the jury is out whether or not I could have handled it as well, but if I had to venture a guess, I'd say NO. In my heart I'll always believe that it was really not my mom, but me they were trying to get away from; someone who steadily held them accountable and was very present. Yes, I had become the Ombudsman from Hell!

TOUR DE NÉCESSITÉ

Two days following the holiday, I found myself, once again, pounding the pavement in search of a new home for Mom. Outside of the odd exception, the majority of facilities that actually had availability were disappointing, to say the least. Perhaps my criterion was bordering on the rigid side, but some of these places were utterly disgusting. Bear in mind, this was all new for me, but I can't even begin to adequately convey my shock at what the marketplace had to offer. Understanding that there was so much more to consider over aesthetics when selecting a facility, my focus had to be redirected. The number one priority at this moment was ensuring that this transition was as seamless as possible.

Upon entering the foyer at selection one, the distinct waft of disinfectant and urine greeted me. Needless to say, my hypersensitive proboscis and I did an about face and hurriedly proceeded to the

next address. Walking into the administration office at location two, another scent-filled greeting
awaited me. Let's name this fragrance "Cigarette
Break." The space was tiny and in total disarray;
papers stacked everywhere. Truly, it looked like an
episode of "Hoarders." That said, the staff members were extremely pleasant, proud of their facility and appeared to really enjoy their work life.
They listened patiently to the saga of JoAnn, and
then began to show me around the living quarters.
All standard offerings are pretty similar in most of
the Alzheimer's buildings. In addition, you often
have the option of a private room, or shared, however, all of the other areas were communal. Yikes!
The Queen just wasn't ready to share a bathroom
and I was not going to force her. What I did leave
with was a new-found knowledge on the difference
between a Private facility and a Medicaid-eligible
property. I'll get into that valuable piece of information a little later.

Visiting dwellings three and four were interesting.
Labeled Adult Family Homes, I wasn't certain what
to expect, but let me see if I can describe them.
The first one was set deep into the woods, away
from the main road. There was no visible security
fencing on the lot, only two older wooded gates
that could be pushed aside by anyone. I couldn't
locate the front porch - only a sliding glass door
on the side of the house. A caregiver answered
the door, but couldn't really provide any details of

the services offered, as the owner was not present. Feeling terribly uneasy anyway, I moved on to the next location.

Adult Family Home two looked like a possibility. There I found a very pleasant Ukrainian family, who had just been granted a license to open their AFH. Their house was clean, spotless in fact, and they were cooking something that smelled amazing. Sorely lacking was any type of security protocol, and in planning for future stages, that type of living situation simply would not suffice.

Arriving at the next address just after 12:30 p.m., I immediately noticed a fire station across the street and saw that the area was being updated. It felt safe enough and I remained hopeful – until the tour began. Entering the family room, I observed nine out of eleven unattended residents slumped over. Albeit at a certain stage it is not uncommon for the neck muscles to become rigid in individuals with Alzheimer's, which contributes to the slumping, it was still disturbing. Missing was any semblance of stimulation, and there were no safeguards in place such as pillows or pads to prevent these poor residents from falling onto each other, not to mention the floor. At her current stage, JoAnn was so full of life, the lack of socialization, or activity in general at this facility, would certainly send her over the edge.

Two more to go before I call it a day; surely I'll find something.   Pulling into the parking lot of number six, a couple of things struck me: 1) the building sat on the edge of a very busy street and 2) it looked very much like an institution, rather than a residence. Convincing myself not to "judge a book by its cover," I ventured inside, with the expectation of being greeted by a receptionist, but there was no one around.   In fact, I walked back and forth down the hallways in search of someone, but not a single soul appeared. My pacing continued for the next twenty five minutes, and still no personnel in sight.   Obviously, it was on to number seven.

Feeling dejected and numb, I walked into the facility and went through the motions. Looking around, it became undeniably clear that I had failed Mom and she would have to settle. Number seven was the worst of them all. Sitting in the lobby, I began to cry and then it happened: God knew I'd had enough and sent an angel to rescue me. The angel was one of the nurses on staff who proceeded to comfort me, while slipping me a piece of paper.   On it was the name of another facility less than ten miles away and their phone number. All she said was "Trust me."

Darkness had set in and I was exhausted, but one last try for Mom wouldn't kill me. Driving into the parking lot, it struck me how closely the building resembled a New England style inn. A black wrought iron fence surrounded the property and the walkway to the entrance was covered by a pretty scalloped awning. There were people on ladders in the process of stringing Christmas lights up onto a large tree outside of the entry and the air was thick with the scent of HoneyBaked Ham. Quite a departure from anything I had seen earlier in the day.

Stepping through the front door and entering the lobby, it looked like a Vermont bed and breakfast; beautifully appointed and decorated for the holidays. The interior of this building was gorgeous! Greeting me with a smile was the receptionist, who promptly phoned for the manager. Within moments, a very pleasant gentleman came over to me, accompanied by his Irish Setter. Overwhelmed and cautiously optimistic, I hit the replay button and told him about JoAnn and recounted my day. He listened patiently and began to share information about their services. In addition to offering Adult Day Care, this facility was divided into Assisted Living, Memory Care for early onset and Memory Care for the later stages. The dining room was the size of a small ballroom, complete with a grand piano in the center, as music was considered a necessary part of each day.

We walked each and every area of the building, including both of the locked and secured wings.

Immensely important to me was observing the staff with their residents after 5:00 p.m. Early evening was often the kickoff of Sundowner's Syndrome (depression, confusion, agitation, increased memory issues, frustration), but to my delight, the only thing I witnessed was a bevy of activity and conversation; there was no evidence of anyone experiencing anything outside of joy. The ratio of staff vs. resident seemed to be two-to-one, although, I'm fairly certain it was the reverse. Still, everyone was looked after, stimulated, and most importantly, seemed genuinely happy. Number eight was a winner!

Now, the last step was to present my findings to the family and hope that we were all in agreement. The only caveat I could see was that this was a private facility, which was not what we were seeking. I had been charged with finding a Medicaid-eligible facility for two reasons: 1) in the event her funds became depleted and 2) we did not wish to move her again should that occur. However, Mom was still functioning at a high level and it was too early in the progression to place her in an environment devoid of interaction.

As mentioned, common practice prior to a new resident moving in is for an assessment to be taken on the individual by a Registered Nurse and a Department Manager. The new facility expeditiously sent their memory care manager over to assess Mom, and, thankfully, through that process it was determined that JoAnn was still capable of living on her own, provided it was within an Assisted Living environment. In total unison, my brother and I submitted the required paperwork and deposits, while preparing Mom for yet another move.

A PERFECT FIT

Moving day arrived, and not a moment too soon! Walking in to my mother's apartment, I found a handful of my dear women friends, already hard at work packing and loading up their cars with Mom's belongings. Unaccustomed to asking for assistance, I was struck by the kindness these ladies displayed, especially without being asked. It was extremely touching and I'll be forever grateful to each and every one of them for as long as I have breath.

Once everything was organized at the latest facility, I picked Mom up and brought her to see her new digs. While she loved the way the apartment looked and adored the building, emotionally, it was quite challenging. The fallout from two moves within thirty days had taken their toll; she was lost, as was any sense of familiarity, essential to the well-being of anyone with Alzheimer's. Visiting her every other day became crucial for the first week, working into every few days, until she was comfortable. At a minimum, I checked in with her by phone daily, as I did not want her to feel lonely, or frightened.

Three weeks into December and everything seemed to be going well. Mom was helping the staff decorate for Christmas, attending all of the socials, and making new acquaintances. That is, until late one afternoon, when my telephone rang. Sometime between breakfast and the lunch hour, Mom went MIA. As she was a highly social creature who couldn't bear missing anything, her caregivers became very concerned when she didn't appear for lunch. A search immediately commenced inside the facility, but as the trail went cold, the investigation moved outdoors. Failing to locate her on the grounds, the frantic search party proceeded outside of the gates where they came upon my confused and coatless mother wandering aimlessly toward a very busy street. Approaching JoAnn with care, the staff made her aware that it was lunchtime. But, Mom explained how she needed to wait outside for her mother and father to pick her up. The fear was that they wouldn't be able to find her inside and she was heading home with them. Mom was gently redirected back to the building by the caregivers and taken directly into the Adult Daycare section, which was locked and secure. Shortly afterwards, she agreed to eat lunch and although no memory of the incident was retained, her intent was still to head home after the meal. Clearly the writing was on the wall; our only viable option now was to place her into Memory Care to ensure her continued safety. You guessed it, I was about to move her again.

Being gregarious and social did not mean that JoAnn wanted a roommate. In fact, she was very unhappy that she no longer had her own apartment. Instead, she was sharing a small space, closet, and a bathroom with a stranger who she was convinced was stealing from her. Ironic, since following that move, JoAnn's wardrobe inexplicably increased by a third and I hadn't spent a dime. With each visit, a new ensemble would present itself, which I came to refer to as The Roommate Collection. Soon I realized that everyone in memory care borrowed from each other and all proprietary control had vanished. Their bedroom doors needed to stay open, and as a result, all apparel was now fair game. No malice was ever behind this behavior, so one learns to accept the situation as the new normal.

Being a fixer, Mom's aversion to sharing a room was hard for me; mostly because I could do absolutely nothing to change the situation. Another serving of tough love had to be administered and that brought to mind something she had repeatedly said to me as a child: "This is going to hurt me more than it's going to hurt you." I didn't ever want to see her unhappy, but this arrangement was in her best interest; and an adept setup it proved to be.

A few weeks after JoAnn was transferred to the secured wing for early stage Alzheimer's (which I refer to as minimum lock-up) and two roommates later, the staff phoned to inform me that she had been moved once again, this time to the maximum security wing. This was an area specifically designated to serve those individuals who had progressed into the later stages of Alzheimer's. Why they felt the need to move her again completely baffled me because she definitely wasn't ready. They quickly explained that in consideration of her obvious desire for additional privacy, Mom would enjoy a larger bedroom in this wing. She would also become the highest functioning resident in her section. That alone made her feel smarter, useful, and somehow back in control. For me, the individuals who were looking after my mom really understood the importance of their work, and I was incredibly grateful.

Going forward, my mother received an abundance of individual attention, met several new people and began to gain back the weight that she'd lost at her previous residence. The caregivers patiently accepted Mom's need to fuss over other residents, understood where the line needed to be drawn, and when redirecting her attention was warranted.

I mean, pushing a wheelchair is one thing, but changing another resident's soiled diaper is entirely different; she couldn't even manage her own.

What you will most likely recognize during the progression of Alzheimer's, is that despite losing the ability to store short-term memories, in a number of cases, the individual may still exhibit traits from their former healthy self. A compelling illustration of this was my mother's instinct for comforting other residents, and attempts to help them execute their daily activities. It was so clear to me that those behaviors directly stemmed from the years she spent working as a registered nurse. Another example that springs to mind is of a gentleman who was residing at the same facility as Mom. Whenever I visited, without fail he would begin a steady vocal recitation of bah-bah-bum, bah-bah-bum. This prompted me to inquire as to whether, or not music had played a part in his past. It did indeed; he was a drummer and his lyrical expression was how he kept time. These discoveries were fascinating and moved me to pay closer attention to the specific characteristics of each inhabitant.

Caregivers who worked for this wonderful organization seemed to have been born of an alternate universe in comparison to others we had previously encountered. Aside from a scant few who were employed at my parents' original Assisted

Living, we hadn't run across anyone who genuinely seemed to appreciate his or her work to the degree that these individuals did. The patience level was off the charts and I assure you, it was not a performance. (Note: Always make it a practice to show up unannounced.) One common theme that continually resonated throughout this facility was that the residents were treated with the utmost respect and would move forward with their dignity intact.

Another notable feature that that stood out was the homey atmosphere. There were even resident pets; a large dog was kept in the early stage Memory Care wing and a cat in the advanced section. Similar to when sharing space with a toddler, these loving creatures patiently endured a daily dose of squeezing, fur pulling, and aggressive petting. Blinded to any loss of mental or physical capability, these loving creatures selflessly offered a highly therapeutic, unconditional affection that became invaluable.

Both the Assisted Living and Memory Care areas maintained separate activity boards, which were rife with regularly scheduled events at all times. Endeavoring to promote stimulation, the activities would include everything from sing-a-longs, board games, spa days (talon clipping and nail polishing), indoor horse racing and Wii tournaments, to piano concerts, comedy shows, and weekly bus rides to the local zoo. The residents were bussed to their various doctor appointments on a bi-monthly basis, as well as taken to the local shops for necessities.

Holidays were especially magical around this fa-cility. Festive decorations, brunches, buffets, and special guests were always a guarantee. Halloween was definitely at the top of my list. One of Mom's favorite caregivers would choose a theme and spend her personal time off in the evenings, self-lessly crafting the most imaginative costumes for the Memory Care tenants. Picture if you will, the Wizard of Oz characters, in a slow and steady pro-cession, sporting wigs, tails, makeup and of course, flanked by their walkers. One tiny woman dressed as the Scarecrow, with hay streaming from her sleeves and pant legs, kept repeatedly proclaim-ing, "I just don't know who I'm supposed to be." Although most of them had no idea what they were doing, they all felt special and included.

The following year, when October 31st rolled around, the same amazing woman created outfits again, this time, in the theme of the Big Top Circus. My mom was artfully transformed into a creative interpretation of a hot air balloon. Suspenders attached to a cardboard box, with both the top and bottom removed became the basket; sun-glasses, a silly hat and a bunch of helium balloons tied to her shirt, completed the look. Once every character was dressed and ready, they formed a line, positioned their walkers and joined the procession through the grand dining room. There they would be judged on their costumes by the other staff members and residents. The visual as a whole was incredibly heartwarming and deservedly so; the Big Top Circus won the contest for their creative attire. Without exception, the fresh environment, coupled with the character of the staff, was in deep contrast to the previous facility. It was truly uplifting to see Mom's metamorphosis; the light had returned to her eyes.

BEFORE THE WELL
RUNS DRY

After a very contented three-year stay, we were com-
pelled to make the difficult decision to move Mom
from the privately funded facility, into one which
was labeled Medicaid-eligible. This was solely out
of necessity and in consideration of her dwindling
finances.

The simple explanation of the difference between Private and Medicaid-eligible is that privately owned and operated facilities are just that.
Because they don't receive funds from the government, residents who exhaust their assets, are
pretty much out of luck and destined to be moved
elsewhere. Perhaps there are a scant few that do
not fit under this umbrella; however, for the most
part, if you can't pay, you cannot stay. Medicaid-
eligible facilities do receive limited supplemental
funding from the government, and therefore, are

able to designate a handful of beds (maybe one or two) as Medicaid-eligible. The requirements are such, that, in order to be qualified for one of those rooms, the resident must reside in that specific facility for no less than two years. Once that requisite period expires, the individual will have the opportunity to be considered, but only if his or her funds are completely depleted and the facility has an available, designated room. Bottomline is that there are no guarantees, which makes the initial decision very difficult.

Like anything else, there are positive aspects and the not-so-positive associated with each. Private facilities are generally nicer and provide much more to a resident in terms of amenities. They are outrageously expensive and should you run out of money, you would be forced to make other arrangements. On the other hand, should you opt for the Medicaid-eligible housing, you'll find fewer offerings for around the same cost, but there is a chance that you could secure a subsidized room if the stars align and you won't have to move your loved one. Basically, it's a gamble with no assurance that you'll be able to stay once the financial well runs dry, but it is an option worth exploring. Assessing where JoAnn sat stagewise, as well as financially, we opted to angle toward the side of just in case and moved her.

The best decision you can make for your loved one is to establish where their cognitive capability lies at this stage in their journey; determine which type of residence most closely meets their personal requirements; spend time evaluating the staff's abilities once you do make your selection; and maintain a clear understanding of their financial portfolio going forward. I realize that with all of the other emotions you must be feeling at this point, it seems crass to be focusing on money, but that's the reality of this situation.

As previously mentioned, we eventually had no choice other than to transfer my mother to a Medicaid-eligible residence, which turned out to be an enormous blessing. The building itself is a small, one-story dwelling and despite the fact that it is solely dedicated to serving those with Alzheimer's and Dementia, it is brimming with more life than any of the other places she had previously inhabited.

Out of the gate, Mom was unsure about everything in her Medicaid-eligible residence, despite being welcomed with open arms by the staff and immediately introduced to a table full of women. Her tightly-wrapped coat remained on and the silence she exuded was deafening. Guilt was the only thing I felt, but somehow this was unlike any of the other moves. Along with the warm, hospitable, and vibrant atmosphere, the caring employees surrounding JoAnn, working overtime to ensure she felt comfortable; I just knew in my heart of hearts, this wasn't a skillful act to impress me; these people were genuine, and my mom would be all right.

The following several months proved me correct. As a result of the facility being so small, it more closely resembled a real home. What it lacked with respect to the accoutrements of a fancier residence, was made up for in spades, by the integrity of the programs in place, the bevy of activities geared toward exercising the mind, and, most importantly, the loving spirit of the team. Prior to this particular move, when visiting my mom, more often than not, I would discover her slumped over and inactive. It was extremely disturbing and made me feel as though she was on a fast track to the end. However, following the move to the Alzheimer's-only facility, the combination of added attention, abundant affection, and increased stimulation ignited a noticeable change in JoAnn. Her Alzheimer's wasn't getting better, but she was becoming increasingly animated and alert.

SEVEN

The seven-stages of decline through Alzheimer's disease is a framework based on a system developed by Dr. Barry Reisberg, Clinical Director of the New York University School of Medicine's Silberstein Aging and Dementia Research Center. Because each individual is of a unique chemical makeup, the rate of progression and the associated behaviors within each stage will vary. There is no such thing as a "One Size Fits All" in any area associated with Alzheimer's disease. What I am offering you in this section are my personal observations as they relate to JoAnn.

Stage 1: No Visible Signs
If there are no signs, why count this as a stage? Because, even though the behaviors seem normal, the disease has established itself internally, and the progression has commenced.

Stage 2: Very Mild
It is difficult to distinguish between Alzheimer's, Dementia and the normal changes attributed to birthdays. Mom's "Skippy" phase presented itself during this period. Initially, it wasn't that noticeable to others; however, the memory issues became more prevalent over the course of a year. Arranging for diagnostic testing was initiated.

Stage 3: Mild
Mom began to experience a noticeable decline in several areas at this juncture. Something as straight-forward as finding an appropriate word for a simple object during a conversation became a struggle, as did her ability to remember where she had put certain things. Straying from her everyday routine became the normal. I recall Mom telling me that she was experiencing a great deal of discomfort in her leg, while simultaneously pointing to her shoulder and saying "Here."

Stage 4: Moderate
Mood swings are very prevalent in this stage. Losing the capability to execute tasks requiring any type of planning, coupled with waning memory retention, pushed her to become withdrawn to a certain extent. In Mom's thinking, it was much easier to stay home than chance embarrassing herself. The deterioration of balance had come into play as well, which is also inherent with aging. It's always

102

unnerving to receive the call about your loved one missing a stair, or falling onto a table. Nowadays, finding JoAnn with bruises here and there unfortunately is commonplace. We did make the decision to buy her a walker, but getting her to accept it was a struggle. That said, it has transformed into her life ring, and, of course, she promptly named it Herkimer.

Stage 5: Moderately Severe
This particular stage was a highly confusing period - for me, anyway. Documentation states that during this period, an individual may no longer be able to recite an address, phone number, or for that matter, the day of the week. But in my mom's case, those symptoms started much earlier. The changes I did notice: Mom now needed assistance with dressing, and, due to the severity of her incontinence, became completely diaper-dependent. We found it exceedingly difficult to take her on outings at this point. Frequently, we would be in a restaurant having a beautiful meal, when she'd have an accident. Without getting graphic, by the time it became noticeable that she needed to be freshened up, it was too late. So often I'd ask her if she needed to visit the Ladies Room and her response would be, "No, thanks – I'm done." If JoAnn had realized what was happening, she would have been mortified! Striving to preserve her dignity, we collectively made the decision to keep Mom close to home. Fortunately, my mother's residence has a designated family dining

room that we can reserve. That affords us the opportunity to bring special occasion meals in to share with her and she feels as though she's dining out.

Because the signs associated with Stage 5 could be mistaken for the traits of a healthy, aging individual, they are often overlooked. In all fairness, without a schedule to follow, one's day can easily run into the next for some and similar to muscles that are not exercised on a continual basis, the brain too, will atrophy.

Stage 6: Severe
Keeping your perspective in check is a must as you navigate through this phase. It is by far one of the most challenging, or at least it has been for me. Mom stopped recognizing me a few years ago, but that is a harsh reality of this juncture; they may stop knowing you. Sleep patterns are turned upside down and wandering at night is not unusual. Toileting, as well as assistance with feeding is commonplace, again, for some. Even though Mom still feeds herself, there have been instances when she expressed confusion related to using the spoon, knife and fork and on occasion, the mechanics of how to swallow. I'll observe my mother trying to eat a green salad with her spoon, or holding a mouthful of juice for twenty seconds before she figures out what to do with it.

Your loved one may also lose the ability to articulate, a condition to which my mother's lovely
caregiver has attached a perfect descriptor, "Word
Salad". JoAnn does her best to say a few words, but
she can't compose a full sentence unless it's gibberish. I respectfully roll with it, and, sensing her
visible frustration, let her know that I understand;
much like you would with a toddler. Then out of
the blue, she swears, clear as day, which as always,
cracks me up. The first time it happened, Mom
was having a hard day. She was trying so hard to
explain something to me, but it was so garbled,
I couldn't figure it out. Visibly upset, I took her
hand in mine and tried my best to comfort her.
Out of nowhere, came a distinct and very audible
expletive. Not much surprises me, but that did. I
turned to her and said, "Are you sure you don't
suffer from Tourette's?" Mom had no idea what
I was talking about, but started giggling and was
instantly redirected to another topic.

The residents at JoAnn's facility are incredibly sweet.
We who choose to visit them regularly are clearly appreciated. Despite the fact that most of the dialogue
is one-sided, the occupants are happy to hold your
hand and listen. My mother stares at me quite a bit
when I'm with her, which leads me to wonder if she's
trying to figure out who I am, or merely being polite
and listening to me. Falling asleep during the conversation happens all of the time as well. Now, bor-
ing has never been an adjective I'd use to describe

myself; perhaps my voice is simply so soothing, it lulls her into a sleep state. Yeah, I'll go with that.

Stage 7: Very Severe
In the final stages of Alzheimer's disease, assistance is needed for almost everything. Notable changes may include the individual ceasing to speak altogether; needing constant help with toileting, feeding and their capacity to swallow disappears. Some experience their muscles becoming so weak that they can no longer hold their heads up. When you find someone slumped over, that is generally the reason. Special wheelchairs are available for those who have reached this juncture. A small cord attached to the top of the wheelchair is hooked to the back of the resident's shirt and should they begin to fall forward, an alarm sounds to alert the caregivers.

Reading through the various stages of decline, you can better understand why each case is unique. Today, my mom sits somewhere between Stages Six and Seven. She smiles, laughs, flirts with the boys (as best she can), walks with her walker, feeds herself, yet is completely incontinent, requires full assistance with toileting, dressing, bathing, and direction. Her balance is diminishing and she falls quite often. Urinary Tract Infections (UTIs) are a regular occurrence. After her move into this wonderful facility, I worked along with the doctor and staff to wean her off of as many medications as we could. Once she made it through the adjustment period, Mom was more alert. Currently, she only takes one in the late afternoon, to curb the symptoms of Sundowner's Syndrome.

Through any given stage, there'll come a time when your loved one will experience Sundowner's. For some reason when the sun is setting, anxiety increases in these individuals with Alzheimer's and Dementia. They may become restless, angry, depressed, frightened, or paranoid. Excessive pacing and hallucinations are also in the mix. As I have stated before, each person is unique and will react differently, but you need to be aware. I have been very blessed, because although Mom occasionally became slightly glum and at times, bitchy, she wasn't violent. The right medication, or as I like to call it, her happy pill, has made a world of difference.

As for the aforementioned UTIs, they are more than simple bladder infections. In the elderly, there are behavioral changes associated with them. Since the individuals are usually unable to communicate what they are feeling, those deportment changes are a great indicator. If left untreated, any infection can accelerate the progression of dementia or Alzheimer's. You simply need to educate yourself on your loved one's patterns and take the appropriate action when warranted.

PERSPECTIVES

My intent with this narrative was to honor my mother in a manner she would respect and appreciate. The knowledge that she perhaps was able to help even one soul through my sharing her stories would make Mom's heart sing. Immeasurable to me is the personal growth and the education I have acquired throughout this journey. To this day, each and every visit with my mother continues to afford me yet another opportunity to observe, not only the changes in her, but the unique manifestation of this disease in the individuals surrounding her. Listening closely to others' accounts of their navigation through Alzheimer's, I became aware of the numerous commonalities inherent with this disease; so numerous in fact, that at times, in discussing certain situations, we could have been speaking about the same person. But it's important to remember that, albeit similar behaviors are exhibited, each individual will react in that person's own unique manner, given a particular circumstance. I cannot stress this enough: A One Size Fits All mentality, does not apply.

Clearly, if you're reading this, you are seeking some fraction of insight about Alzheimer's disease and what you can expect. Following Mom's initial diagnosis, I wish I'd been provided the opportunity to read about other people's experiences with Alzheimer's and tap into their reality; it definitely would have been of tremendous comfort.

The best advice I can propose is as follows: At the exact moment you step across the threshold of your loved-one's residence, "buckle up." You will have entered their realm and despite what one may believe, it is not an environment to fear. In fact, within some of the goings-on we might find unusual, there lies a silent grace. Most of the people I have encountered with the disease are sweet, gentle, and completely unaware of their condition. They endeavor to engage me in a dialogue and occasionally during a visit, I feel them stroke my hair, or my shoulder. Something about me must seem familiar or comfortable to them, which makes me smile. From the tiny grandma sporting different hats each day with her purse around her forearm, to the woman sharing tea with a propped up photo of her deceased husband, their world is one that I have elected to respect and embrace. These are perfect examples of individuals with Alzheimer's displaying characteristics of their former selves. When they do, it is truly beautiful to witness.

You are the only one in control of your take away from these visits. They are important to the loved one, because you are giving your special person your time and attention, but trust me; down the road these visitations are going to be immensely valuable to you. I rather enjoy my dropping in to see Mom, especially when I'm in the market for a shoulder to cry on. There's nothing better than having a private dialogue with someone, knowing fully well that it will stay private. Guaranteed within thirty seconds, there will be no retention with respect to my visit, let alone the conversation. Mom remains my safe place, best friend, and the ultimate, personal "vault."

There have also been moments that I consider to be gifts. On Mother's Day earlier this year, I was visiting JoAnn and relaying a story. She began to look at me very strangely and all of a sudden, burst into tears. Cupping my face in her hands, which incidentally was in her repertoire of signature moves, she repeatedly said, "I love you, I love you, I love you." Fifteen seconds later, I once again resumed my role as the "sweet girl who visits." It may have been Mother's Day, but it was I who received a gift.

The information I have offered is my truth, born from my experiences with JoAnn. Should you, the reader, be able to strike a connection with one of the accounts, you'll quickly realize you're not in this alone. Let me pose a question: On those occasions where you find yourself needing to repeat something fifteen times within the same conversation, how does that actually affect your existence? I'll answer for you – it doesn't! Yes, it can be exasperating, but in the end, you are really only being asked for a little time and patience.

Above all else, remember this is NOT ABOUT YOU! Be mindful that you are dealing with an illness and if you change YOUR perspective, you'll be better equipped to handle what comes.

WHERE'S MY PURSE?

Alzheimer's disease is tricky, namely because of the ebb and flow. All right, tricky may not be an accurate adjective. Perhaps a more appropriate descriptor is frustrating. There are points in time when you are convinced, beyond a reasonable doubt, that the disease has reversed itself. You want so badly for life to return to normal and your loved one to get better. But what you really need to ask yourself is "for whom?" It isn't about us and our loved ones aren't aware. Mom changed and I adapted, by altering my perspective and accepting the gracious oblivion of her new world.

Admittedly, I can be a bit of a Pollyanna. In the past, I've been described as "a little too positive," to which I'd reply, "It's my bubble and I'm happy in it." Now don't get the wrong impression; we all have our moments, but giving in to self-pity, at least where my mom is concerned, isn't an option for me. As well, it is my belief that one's choice of optimism should be applauded, not ridiculed. Scores of creditable writings are available from self-help gurus, which characterize us as being either a "glass half full" or "glass half empty" type. My perspective steers me in a different direction; making the absolute most out of what I am presented. The glass in front of me will always contain the appropriate amount.

"Where's my purse?" was a query my mom posed to us on a continual basis. It became a ribbing point that the family thoroughly enjoyed teasing her about, as it happened so frequently. Some days the intervals could be as close as five minutes apart. Ordinarily, all she needed to do was reach down next to her chair to retrieve it, yet she still asked. Similar to most women, that handbag carried Mom's life support, meaning her lipstick, eyeliner, hankies, rain bonnet, keys, wallet, breath mints, assorted photos, and of course, hidden money. Honestly, she had so much loot tucked away in every little pocket of the purse, we nicknamed it the Bank of JoAnn. Her theory behind distributing the cash around the bag was if someone should steal it, he or she wouldn't be able to locate all of the dough. Once again, an admirable, yet flawed thought process. She remained constantly on guard and we taunted her relentlessly, all with love and entirely in jest.

One thing that to this day remains true - Mom can laugh, especially at herself. She's no longer able to articulate a full sentence, nor does she understand everything I say to her. But during our little dates, we laugh and hold hands. The knowledge that I'm her daughter has faded, but somehow we are still connected. I am my mother's purse: A mere shell filled with her inherent characteristics and values; everything she has so closely guarded throughout my existence. She needn't ever worry about where I am, because the answer will always be the same - forever by her side.

EPILOGUE

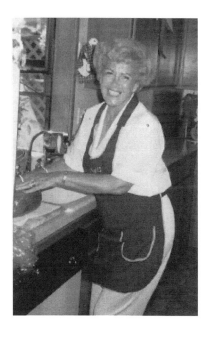

I completed my mother's story in January of 2014. Shortly thereafter, on March 8, 2014, Mom began her new life in Heaven with a healthy mind, a lively spirit and a huge smile.

PART TWO

RECOLLECTION

CHRISTINE

Today I went to the cemetery to see my mom, clean off the headstone and take her some flowers for Thanksgiving. It has been almost two years since she passed away from that terrible disease Alzheimer's. She was diagnosed in 2001 and spent the last thirteen years with it, which was shocking to me. The good news is that she did not suffer at all, and we were also very fortunate to have found great medical care from the onset. Various Alzheimer's medications were administered in an effort to halt the disease, but sadly, they were unsuccessful. It's amazing that with all of the progress scientists have made in medicine, this terrible disease has not yet been eradicated!

My mom, Christine, was born in Piraeus, Greece in 1927. She lived a very happy life there and was blessed to have attended a great school. When she turned sixteen, her father made the decision to move to America, to establish a new life for his family. Prior to leaving themselves, my uncle, mother, and grandmother made a trip to the Horyo to say goodbye to members of their extended family. Shortly after their arrival, the war broke out and tragedy ensued. My uncle was killed at the hands of the Germans, which led Mom and YaYa (my grandmother) to remain there for the next two years.

Because her father was already in the States, he was able to get money to them through the Red Cross, but it did little good, as there was not much to buy. The original plan was a short two-day stay, so all of their winter clothing was still in Piraeus. My mother had no warm clothes or shoes with her, so her uncle, one of the family members she had gone to visit, made her a pair of wooden shoes lined with leather to keep her feet warm. No, none of them had planned on spending the entire season there, let alone two years.

Once the war ended, she and her mother left for America and finally settled in Seattle, where her father lived. There, they truly began their life in the states; Mom enrolled in school, obtained her driver's license, and became a citizen. My grandfather continued to bring the rest of his siblings over to join them, ensuring that my mom would be surrounded by many cousins and family members.

Attending Greek dances was one of Mom's favorite things to do and that is where she met my father, the love of her life. He served in the Navy, but returned to the University of Washington to complete the Interior Design program and obtain his degree. After his graduation, they moved to Portland, Oregon where he worked as a designer at a local furniture store and I was born. Our family resided there for one year, but following the death of my grandfather, we returned to Seattle, where Dad would oversee and manage the family restaurant. My mom helped out as needed, even though she was pregnant with her second child. Sadly, my sister was born with a hole in her heart, in addition to a cleft palate, and she passed away after only two months, leaving Chris devastated.

Chris immersed herself in activity and became very involved in the Greek Church bazaars. An avid cook, she contributed a lot of the baking for the pastry booth, looked after the Milk fund, participated in the Children's Hospital Guild, and acted as PTA president. She was an amazing entertainer and could whip up a gourmet meal in minutes! Flowers were another love of Mom's and it was obvious to everyone who knew her. She could grow anything and her flower arrangements were gorgeous! My mother was such a kind individual and was willing to do anything for anyone. In fact, after I gave birth to my first child, my parents couldn't get enough of her. This was fortunate for us, because our house was on the market and sold faster than we had anticipated, leaving us with no option other than to move in with them. We stayed there until we bought another home, which probably was too soon for Mom & Dad, as they loved having my daughter around.

Fall settled in and my parents planned a trip to New England with their best friends to see the changing foliage. My dad began feeling ill, so Mom insisted he visit the doctor before they left. The outcome of that visit was something neither of them had expected; he was diagnosed with pancreatic cancer and died two months later. Dad's death took a devastating toll on both my mother and my daughter. It wasn't until three years later, when I gave birth to my second daughter, that the spark returned to Mom's eyes. We were thankful that she had a number of wonderful friends with whom; she did a lot of traveling. But that said, she was never quite the same after losing my dad.

The first sign of Alzheimer's presented itself ten years later. If I'm being completely honest, I had actually observed a few things that were amiss during the six months prior, but now others were beginning to notice. Apparently, my mom had planned to cook dinner for some family friends, and, in the process, suddenly turned on all of the burners simultaneously and became extremely disoriented. Naturally, I was called, as they had no idea what was happening. Making up excuses seems to be a common response in this type of situation, which is exactly what I found myself doing. I picked Mom up and brought her home with me, where I knew she'd be safe. Then I promptly scheduled an abundance of medical testing. Watching her struggle to put the time on the clock during the Clox testing was painful and made me cry. She had become my child and I wasn't allowed to help her with the test.

Residing in our home was short-lived. Because there was always a great deal of activity in our house, Chris was very unhappy. Also challenging was the fact that I couldn't leave her by herself, so I ended up taking her everywhere with me. In the meantime, I tried to find a caregiver who could stay with Mom in her own home, but that proved to be a tall order. After interviewing an excess of individuals, I did find a suitable candidate; however, it didn't work out. We tried two more times, until I came to the realization that I was spending more of my time babysitting the caregivers than they were spending looking after Mom. My daughter, Jayme, offered up her weekends to provide some time off to the live-ins. She would actually climb into the shower with Chris to shave her legs and bathe her, then dress Mom up and take her out to lunch. The compassion my daughter displayed was amazing and made my mother very happy. It would have been wonderful to find an adult caregiver that had as much character as Jayme.

Continuing to visit a couple times each week, I still wasn't satisfied with the level of care Mom was receiving, and some items had gone missing. So my next quest was to get her into a nursing home, which was easier said than done. After touring twenty-three homes, I decided on a facility in Bellevue, close to my home. It was a nice, comfortable environment with none of the typical odors that one might associate with similar environments, and the staff took great care of my mom. They had a beauty shop where she could have her hair and nails done, as well as a loaded Activities calendar. This included fashion shows, cooking, baking, gardening and cocktail hours! All the things she loved were right under the same roof and the quality of care she was receiving made me happy.

The time came when Mom lost the ability to speak. Albeit there was really no conversation going on, I would still go three times each week to see her, which provided me the opportunity to get to know the caregivers. I can't be certain, but it's possible that may have helped to get my mother even better care.

Six years later, we decided it was time to move her into a Home Care facility, which was five minutes

from my home. On my way to work each morning, I was able to take leftovers and Greek cooking
to Mom. During my visits now, I would color her
hair, paint her nails and give her pedicures. I'd
buy her cute sweats, slippers and spend time with
her either watching TV, or just sitting. She started sleeping a lot more and began to visibly lose
weight, but her health was still good. Even though
she was completely non-verbal, Mom appeared to
be unaware and content. I had accepted that she
was "gone" eight years before now, but her decline
was still very slow and frustrating; this was not how
my mom would want to live. My Dad's mother
had Alzheimer's, so I had been through this exercise before. One thing I clearly remember my
mother telling me is if she ever was diagnosed with
Alzheimer's disease, "shoot her." Obviously, that
was not going to happen, but I understood, because she wasn't really living a life she would have
chosen.

Mom peacefully passed away in her sleep and I
miss her every day. But, I know in my heart she is
exactly where she should be - with my dad and the
rest of her family! I love you Mom!

Georgi Stocker

POP

This story is dedicated to my wonderful mother. She did not suffer from dementia, or Alzheimer's, but my stepfather developed a form of dementia after Mom's passing. They loved each other so very much and it is my belief that following her death, the loneliness was too much for him, which led him to lose his purpose.

My mother had been married to my biological father for forty-nine years when he passed away. For her, it felt as though an entire lifetime had transpired. After a significant amount of time had gone by, my three sisters and I encouraged Mom to find new friends and that included a possible suitor. She was still a pretty, vibrant woman at age 68, and we were solely focused on her happiness going forward.

Well, it finally happened; Mom met someone. The new man was ten years her junior and had a few health problems; however, they were a perfect pair. You may be wondering if the family had any concerns about this union, but it was quite the opposite. All anyone needed to do was to observe them as a couple, cuddling and having so much fun planning their new life, and one couldn't help but know "it was meant to be," and that it was!

Pop, as we called him, was very good at fixing things, as well as working with wood. He made a nice home for our mother and spoiled her. Her wish was his command; when she asked for a new shelf to put her teacups on, voila, a new white shelf appeared. He also loved surprising her with thoughtful gifts, such as homemade wood planters for her flowers. She had quite a flair for placing furniture, lamps, tables, and memorable photographs in just the right place, and together with Pop's woodworking skill, they were a perfect pairing.

As expected in getting older, the two of them were experiencing a few health problems, but in general, they were doing quite well. A change was in the air, though. One day while visiting, we noticed that Pop was becoming somewhat irritated. This was very out of character for him, as he was usually very engaging, so it caused us some concern. If we said anything, Mom, always his greatest supporter, would quickly come to his defense, stating that he was either not feeling well, or worried about something. Even though he enjoyed seeing the family, I think he was happier when it was just the two of them. During the twenty years they were together, my mother and Pop were rarely apart and it seemed stressful for him when there were too many people around; he wasn't comfortable with change.

My dear, sweet mom was the most loving and caring person. She would always know just what to say, and when language would slant in a critical direction, she'd deliver it in a funny way, sticking to her point, while making us laugh. We always understood why Pop loved her so, and after she passed away, we were all left incredibly sad.

In the days immediately following Mom's passing, we gathered together to reminisce and console each other. In an effort to be sensitive and thoughtful with all four of us, Pop gave us the opportunity to choose whatever precious mementoes of Mom's we wished to keep. However, that was short-lived. Not long after we had gone back home and he had been alone for a while, my stepfather began making snap decisions with little regard for anyone else. Erratically, he started to dispose of everything by selling my mother's clothes, furniture, and finally, their home. This wasn't a matter of his simply wanting to move on; we soon realized that he was beginning to lose touch with reality.

No longer able to live alone, Pop went to live with his son. He had always wanted to one day begin fishing and hunting again, but sadly, that didn't happen. His behavioral changes became more apparent and the new living situation was not meeting his expectations. Loneliness was increasing, as was his negativity, and soon, one problem led to another. The only option left for him was to be placed in an Assisted Living environment, where hopefully, he would be less lonely in the company of others.

Once you move your loved one into an Assisted Living, you develop an overwhelming sense that you somehow have left them alone and isolated. Ideally, you would like to visit often and help them through the adjustment period. In our case, however, that simply was not possible because he lived far away. When we were able to see him, it became quite apparent that Pop was unhappy and wanted to leave. Collectively, the family agreed to move him again.

Moving a parent from one state to another, in addition to getting approval for facility and medical changes can be stressful for all parties. This is especially true, if you cannot be certain that this change will improve your parent's circumstances. That said, you love them and have to do something. At this point, I kept thinking of my mom and how this man took such great and loving care of her for so many years. We knew in our hearts that her wish would be for her girls to do whatever it took to ensure that he was safe and happy.

As you might have guessed, the move did not make things better for anyone. No matter how nice his room was, or how many social opportunities were presented, it seemed impossible to engage him. Eventually, unless forced, Pop wouldn't shave, or shower, and no longer cared how he looked. Becoming increasingly weak and afraid, he had basically checked out.

On several occasions we were summoned to his side after he was rushed to the hospital with a diagnosis of breathing problems. Miraculously, he was feeling good as new upon our arrival and very happy to see us. During another visitation, we noticed that a few key essentials he had asked us to bring him had gone missing. We later uncovered that his dentures, shaver, wallet, radio, and various framed photos had been tossed over a fence outside of his room, into a deep ravine where we could not retrieve them. When asked why he discarded these items, Pop could offer no explanation.

It became very clear to us, that although we had placed him into an environment which was safe, happy and social, it would never be his home, or enough to address his broken heart. The Assisted Living doctor concluded that Pop should undergo a mental health evaluation, as he was now stating that he no longer wanted to live. We were optimistic when taking him in to be evaluated and hopeful that upon diagnosis, a treatment could be administered. This evaluation turned out to be quite the eye-opener for the family. His doctor was completely upfront with him and spoke freely to the realities of the situation; something that we were reluctant to do ourselves. All of this was new territory for us as well.

Heading back to the Assisted Living facility was a challenge. Pop was seated on the passenger side of the car and repeatedly kept reaching for the door handle, as though his plan was to open it and jump out. I finally pulled off to the side of the road, and exasperated, asked him what he was doing. Silence was his only response. The child safety lock was employed for the remainder of the trip.

Eventually, the time came when we had to move Pop into a group home. The family who operated the home was very nice. We visited often, took him on several short outings, and out to dine on fish and chips, which was his favorite! Then one day we got a call to say that he had broken the window shades and tried to leave the home, which, we were informed, was not the first time. He was no longer in control of himself; the dementia was driving his behavior.

Visits to the hospital became more frequent for Pop near the end. He would become very ill, but after a week of hospitalization and non-stop attention, the marked improvement would send him home. During Pop's last hospital stint, his son came to visit and ultimately, made the decision to take his dad back home with him for the duration. That made my stepfather and the family very happy. We said our goodbyes and on the journey home, he passed in his sleep.

It is so difficult losing your loved ones. With respect to Pop, I'm confident that all of us did our very best, by caring for and loving him with all of our hearts. We continue to think of both him and my mother together, which helps to bring us a little peace. I love you, Mom.

P.S. Pop, thank you for taking such great care of her!

P.O.

ALBERT

My father was born in Ohio in 1914. He was one of twelve children and the baby of the family. Growing up in an ethnic neighborhood with little money, he and his family led a very simple life. Their days were spent working very hard, so in the evenings they could relax with friends and family. Most of the family members were musically inclined and played an assortment of instruments. So during these get-togethers, the entire family would play music, in addition to enjoying homemade food and various wines they had produced.

Dad was a professional musician who taught himself to play banjo, guitar and accordion, beginning at the age of twelve. Similar to most entertainers, he was a very outgoing, happy, and lovable man. He was full of vitality and spent much of his time teaching music to young adult students, honing his craft. During the hours he wasn't teaching, my dad could be found working on many projects around the house, or playing golf, while still working in the evenings as an entertainer. Also on the resume was the four-year term he served in the First Armored Division in both Africa and Italy during World War II. Following the end of the war, he married my mother and together they had three children.

The relationship between my father and me was close. I looked up to him and admired his good looks, talent and warm personality. When I was very young, he indulged me by playing a game we called "Barbershop", where I'd comb his hair and pretend to shave him until he fell asleep on the sofa. As a musician, he was continually practicing his instruments, as well as recording sound tracks for his work. He would let me sit with him to observe, which I thoroughly enjoyed. Shortly after I was married, I moved out of state. Due to the distance, we were no longer able to spend the amount of time together that we had in the past, and I felt sad about that.

Memory problems began to surface for my dad in his late 60's. He had always been prone to misplacing his keys or glasses, but now he had begun to forget a few additional things. At the time, I attributed this to nothing more than aging. But, as Dad moved into his early to mid-70's, he began forgetting more serious things for instance, that he had put water on to boil, what he had gone to the store to purchase and more notably, he couldn't remember how to play a particular song that he had been playing for years. For a brief while, we believed these concerns might have been linked to his hearing loss, but a bigger blow was forthcoming. My dad had to discontinue working because he could no longer remember how to play his music.

Over time, Dad became less communicative when the family would congregate. As well, it became hurtful to me when he would not engage in play with my young son. I continued to tell myself it was related to his hearing loss. Because I had moved away with my husband when Dad was in his early 60's, I missed out on much of the controversy about his health that was taking place back home. His memory loss was apparent to us only when we visited, because we did not see him that often. Despite my minimum exposure to Dad's cognitive changes, I was still very concerned.

My mom did not want to acknowledge the fact that my dad was having increasing memory difficulties. When I tried to mention the facts to her, she perpetuated the idea that Dad's hearing problems were the main cause of his memory loss; perhaps that's where I picked up that idea. Mom and Dad were the children of immigrants and, as such, had been raised with the belief that health, finances and any other matters of a personal nature were not to be discussed with anyone, including their adult children. This belief, unfortunately, put a great strain on my mom. It also prevented my dad from getting the proper medical attention until after her passing, when he was eighty.

Once Mom passed away, Dad's health deteriorated rapidly. I spent a week with him after Mom's funeral and was shocked to see how serious his health had become. One evening Dad and I went out for dinner and he insisted on driving. I became very frightened, as he almost caused two accidents and could not remember how to get to the restaurant, which was less than one mile away. At that point, I told my sister, who still lived in the same town with him, that we needed to take away his car keys.

Stripping my father of his driving privileges proved to be a huge obstacle, and he was extremely unhappy with us. The only way my sister was able to convince Dad to agree that he could no longer drive, was to have his doctor back up our recommendation. Once we had the physician's collaboration, we would simply remind him that it was Doctor's orders when he wanted to get behind the wheel. It was also at this time that we received a formal diagnosis; his condition was definitely Alzheimer's disease. The doctor immediately started him on an Alzheimer's medication and a significant improvement was noted with his memory; but it certainly was not a cure.

Since Dad was having a difficult time running the house, we decided to bring a caregiver in to assist him. The woman we hired did the cooking, cleaning, ran errands, and helped Dad get out of the house a bit. This worked well for a very short time, until the neighbors began to notice my father wandering the streets of the neighborhood, completely lost. We knew that it was time to move him into an Assisted Living apartment. No surprise, Dad was very opposed to this idea. He did not want to leave his home of forty plus years. We did our best to sell him on all of the benefits a move into an Assisted Living would provide: his meals would be prepared; his apartment would be cleaned; and laundry would be done. Finally, after a lot of convincing, he reluctantly gave in. The family was pleased that Dad adjusted rather well following the move, especially when he met a woman who looked amazingly similar to my mother. They were quick to form a romantic relationship, which shocked the nurses. My sister and I responded, "Way to go, Dad!"

Everything seemed to be working out well for a few short months, until my father figured out how to exit a back door at the facility. He was found wandering the streets of the city by some policemen. We then moved him to an Alzheimer's facility with separate cottages for each level of the disease. Dad was never very happy in this residence, but at least we knew he was well cared for and safe. Initially, he sat in an earlier stage of the disease, so was not quite as advanced as most of the other individuals in his cottage. When he'd witness other residents' temper outbreaks, or conversations with themselves, he thought they were crazy. That alone made him want to leave and return home, but we continually reminded him that his house had been sold and this was home.

As the disease progressed, Dad had to be moved to different cottages within the facility. Although he remained safe, clean and well fed, he was never happy. Hallucinations began, which led him to believe he was on a train that he needed to exit. While visiting my father, I observed the desperation in him to get off of that imaginary train and I would do anything possible to try and calm him down.

Eventually, he lost the ability to communicate with me. After some time had passed, I chose to discontinue calling him, as the one-sided conversations were proving too difficult to continue. Instead, I began writing letters to my father. Advancing into the next stage, Dad went through a very emotional period. The worst experience I can recall was the time he began to cry when I was leaving and continued to do so for over twenty four hours. It was devastating.

Throughout the ten years my dad was living in a facility, there was little humor, much sadness and frustration. There was also, an abundance of thankfulness to all the men and women who cared for him on a daily basis.

Albeit not often, there was on occasion, something that struck us funny. An instance that comes to mind is one that my brother-in-law related to me and it still makes me chuckle. There was a woman living in the cottage with my dad, who routinely wandered around throughout the day muttering "I hate this f—ing place, I hate this f—ing place, I hate this f—ing place." One day my brother-in-law got tired of hearing her repetitive statements and said, "I think this is a very nice place, don't you?" The woman answered whole-heartedly, "Yes, I do." Immediately, she resumed her pacing and began to mutter once again, "I hate this f—ing place!"

It has been nearly ten years since my dad's long journey with Alzheimer's ended and for that, I am thankful. He was ill for close to twenty years, which is a very long time to live with this disease. Unfortunately, Alzheimer's ran in his family and three of his brothers also were diagnosed and later died because of it. My father's death brought relief to our family, with the knowledge that he was no longer suffering. I still miss him and feel very nostalgic every time I pass his picture in my hallway. But, I know he is in a good and happy place, together with my mom.

Having traveled this path with my dad has made me a more compassionate and understanding person, particularly with the sick and elderly. I have become more spiritual in many ways, as well. Maybe this, too, is a sign of my own aging (the dreaded word!), but I hope and pray that God spares me from the same terrible fate that my father, like so many others, has suffered through.

My husband and I are avid supporters of the Alzheimer's Association and hope that a cure is found soon. With my family history, we may need the cure someday in the fairly near future.

Anonymous

ERNIE

It's funny, at the ripe old age of fifty four, which memories are still fresh for me.

My dad, Ernie, was a boxer. I remember as a little girl, going to the ring with him and watching him and his pals spar. In fact, Dad was a Featherweight champ at one time, and I have the poster to prove it! Another thing about my father, he was a drinker. Back in his day, he owned several bars, so we accepted it as being something that "goes with the territory."

I still have memories of our outings with Ernie. He used to take my brother and me on car rides that would entail our moving from bar to bar. We would sit and wait patiently in the car for my father to come out. Eventually, when he did reappear, it would be with a friend in tow, who would proceed to fawn over us with "oohs" and "aahs", remarking on how grown up we'd become. Disappointing, because the only thing my brother and I really wanted to do was spend time with our dad. The best part of those driving adventures for us was listening to him sing silly songs and, every once in a while, curse at the driver in the car next to his. He was a very funny guy!

Dad's job of buying and selling bars eventually led him to move so far away from us, we were only able to see each other once or twice each year. Since our time with my father was so limited, we did not see the gradual change in him, or notice that he was losing his sense of self. This change became apparent, as well as scary for us, on those occasions when we did get together.

A decision was made by my brother, to venture across the country to pack Ernie up and then bring him home. I was pregnant, but spent my days taking my dad to various doctor's appointments. We were fortunate that he was a veteran, because all of his life savings were now gone and he was undergoing multiple tests. The test results only confirmed what we already knew: Dad had Alzheimer's disease, although, the doctor stated that they could never be completely sure.

Following the birth of my son, my father would sing him the songs he used to sing to me. He was so very sweet to my little boy. But challenges soon started presenting themselves. A particular day comes to mind when I arrived home to find an extremely irate husband. Apparently, my father had attempted to reheat something and nearly burned our house down. On another occasion, I received a call from a sweet woman at a local fast-food restaurant. She asked me if I knew a man named Ernie, to which I replied, "Yes, he's my father." Evidently, he had become a bit disoriented, so he wandered inside and asked the lady to phone me. Immediately, I was on my way, but when I got there, no one had any inkling of the incident. Quickly, I figured out that the fast-food restaurant this woman phoned me from was twelve miles away. My dad took many walks; I believe it was what he did to fill the time and feel some sense of purpose. One day he walked from my house in Laurelhurst to his brother's in West Seattle – approximately, thirteen miles. I remember looking over his tattered shoes after that and being amazed at his determination. Soon, I came to the realization that my dad's days of living with us were numbered.

Finally, the time arrived when it was necessary to move my father into an environment that provided more safety. I cried when we had to tell him. Although he had his own room and a bit of freedom, he did not want to be there. Eventually, after making some new friends, he was able to settle in. It's amazing what a strong tool the mind can be when paired with one's instinct to survive. Dad was convinced that he had a job and a girlfriend, which improved his demeanor. The only thing that mattered to us was that he remained safe and happy, so whatever he wanted to imagine was fine. Sadly, his stretch of contentment ended. In defending his pretend girlfriend, Ernie took a swing at another resident and if that wasn't enough, he wandered away yet again, boarded a bus, and got lost. With those behaviors, my dad bought himself a ticket to a locked ward.

Going forward, I visited my father as often as possible. During those visits, we would dance together, as it seemed that music was the only thing he could remember at this stage. Gone was any recollection of my identity; however, he could hum the tune of "Brown Eyed Girl" with no effort. I'd often stare into his eyes, searching for some type of recognition, and on occasion, convince myself that I'd witnessed a connection. Admittedly, I believe it was my way of coping with the loss.

Dad passed away at the age of seventy-six, which is the current age of my mother who still runs around Green Lake. I'm really not certain which parent I will grow to resemble, but I do know the sparkle in my eye and the tune of my voice were inherited from my dad.

Kathy Davis Hayfield

ISABELLE

I would like to introduce you to my mother-in-law, Isabelle. She has dementia and was officially diagnosed in 2005, after her loving husband of nearly sixty-five years passed away.

Mom, as I refer to her, was born in Fresno, California in 1920 and at the age of two, moved with her family to Detroit, Michigan. This is where she would spend her youth and attend school before moving back to Fresno in 1939. Isabelle was a good student and excelled in all subjects. As well, she played the piano and loved to participate in sports. My mother-in-law always enjoyed sharing tales of her childhood adventures in Detroit with me and was reportedly labeled the resident "tomboy" by her family and friends.

The family was a very large, closely-knit one with many of the aunts, uncles and cousins living in Detroit. Mom loved going on about her times spent at the shared family cottage on the lake and all the fun she had with her cousins, which were very fond memories for her.

In 1939 Isabelle, her father, mother and two sisters, moved back to Fresno. That is where she met and fell in love with my father-in-law, George. They married in 1941 and had three sons, one of whom is my husband, Kenneth. Theirs was a solid, stable marriage, dedicated to the family, as well as the responsibility of the family business: ranching in the central valley of California. Mom loved all of us more than anything, and took great pride in raising her sons and making a comfortable home for them.

Ken and I married in 1972, which is the day I became a part of this wonderful family and have remained so for close to forty years. During that span, Mom and I developed a loving, caring relationship. In fact, I respect and love her as though she were my own mother. My husband and I have two children, the first two of five grandchildren for my in-laws. Mom's first great grandchild, our granddaughter, is now fourteen months old. Family continues to be everything to her.

My father in-law suffered a stroke at the age of seventy eight and it was following that event, when we first noticed that Mom was having problems. She started experiencing bouts of depression, and dealing with Dad's medical issues was proving to be very difficult for her. Eventually, she became more withdrawn and started to isolate herself from family and friends. The confusion and forgetfulness became more apparent, but sadly, the seriousness of her condition went unnoticed for some time.

Living several hours away did not afford my husband or me the opportunity to witness the day-to-day progression and deterioration. Our thought was that, as my father-in-law's health continued to improve, Mom would get better. Thankfully, his health did recover and life seemed pretty much back to normal. But while he had returned to his former schedule of spending his days at the office or on the golf course, Isabelle's condition worsened. She spent her days at home, becoming increasingly more isolated, ceasing to maintain her home, and stopping all cooking and cleaning. Another sure sign for us was that she began to let her personal appearance decline. Always very fussy about how she presented herself to others, we knew something was wrong when she started cancelling her standing, weekly hair appointments.

Due to Mom's symptoms being attributed to depression, the gradual changes were overlooked. Ken's brothers lived nearby and saw her several times each week. They would report back to us that Mom was depressed and refusing to take her medication, so for a very long time, that explanation sufficed. I'm not assigning any blame, as we were all in the dark about what was really transpiring. No one was aware how serious this had become, nor how to approach the issues. Mom's doctors at the time were not much help to us either. Misdiagnosing her in the earlier stages only delayed an intervention and proper treatment.

Throughout the first year after my father-in-law's death, Isabelle remained in her home. My brothers-in-law would check on her several times during the day and provide her with her meals etc. For the overnight hours we hired a care-giver who would spend the evening, arriving at around 8:00 p.m. and leaving in the early morning. This was not an ideal solution, as Mom was really unhappy about having strangers in her home. She was also convinced this person was stealing from her and trying to hurt her. The decline continued and after several months of battling indecision on the next steps and still without a firm diagnosis of dementia, we knew something had to be done. Without my father-in-law to take care of her, it was clear that she was in trouble and could no longer live on her own.

The retirement facility we chose only had an opening for a semi-private room in Skilled Nursing. We reluctantly agreed to take the space, with the guarantee that as soon as an opening for a private room in Assisted Living became available, she would be moved. This was a really sad and emotional time for all of us. No family wants to have to make the kinds of decisions we were faced with. Initially in the first several weeks, Mom was very unhappy, however, once she got to know her caregivers and became more comfortable in her surroundings, things changed. A few months passed and an Assisted Living room opened up, so we moved her again. It took less than two weeks in her new apartment for our reality check; Mom was much worse than we had originally thought and needed to be in a secured setting.

Isabelle's doctors were now prescribing three separate medications; an antidepressant and two additional drugs for her dementia. In the months that followed, many adjustments to her medications and the respective dosages needed to be made. Some days she would appear heavily drugged and sleep around the clock, while other days Mom was alert, agitated and combative. The side effects of the medicines also came into play, as they had a tendency to produce terrible nightmares and hallucinations. Modifications to her drug regimen in search of the proper mix were an ongoing process. Outside of the dementia, Mom is very healthy and for that we are grateful. That said, it is of ongoing concern to the family that Isabelle is sleeping most of each day, possibly due to the medication.

Five years have gone by and my mother-in-law still asks "Why she is here?" and "When she is going home?" Now and again, you may hear Isabelle comment that they take great care of her and that she likes her new home. No longer does Mom inquire about her house or about my father-in-law. What she does love to revisit are very early memories of her life and childhood. If asked specific questions regarding her family, or things she did as a child, Mom does seem to remember and can recount with a large degree of detail. Other memories Isabelle can speak of are the time when she and my father-in-law first met, their wedding, his time in the military, and the war. When my father-in-law was away in the military, Mom lived with her own widowed father and has plenty of tales to share about that period. But if you asked her what she had for lunch ten minutes ago, she would not be able to tell you. There would be no recall of lunch, period!

In some ways, the fact that Mom had dementia during her husband's death may have been a blessing. The short term memory loss seemed to act as a buffer for the pain of losing her beloved partner, although at the time, we were not aware that the disease had advanced to that degree.

I feel extremely blessed to have this wonderful lady in my life. She is a truly loving, nurturing and caring person and everyone who has ever known Isabelle, loves her. Full of personality, effervescent, with a great wit and sense of humor; to this day when we talk, something very silly can set off the giggles with us. Thank God the disease hasn't taken that away!

Our children are also very blessed to have this special lady to call grandmother and each of us holds dear many wonderful, fond memories of times spent with Mom and Dad. Excitement would always build around the anticipation of the upcoming visits, which were truly a time of celebration for us. Residing inside each individual's heart are unique and loving memories of times shared with their grandparents. Recently, we organized a mini-family reunion with Mom and were able to spend an entire afternoon visiting her. She had a good time with her children and grandchildren and I recognized that familiar look of contentment in her eyes. Knowing the entire family was together brought joy to her, if only for a short while.

Mom will not get better; she will always have dementia, this insidious thief of one's very being. "Dear Lord, please keep Isabelle safe and free of pain. Know that we are grateful for the good years, as well your guidance in creating the loving and special memories that we will forever cherish."

Chris - February 13, 2012

Dear Mom,

Thank you for loving me and making me feel like your daughter and a part of the family. Also, thank you for being such a special and loving grandmother to our children. They will always hold dear the many memories of times spent with Grandma and Grandpa.

As my mind sweeps back over the last forty-two years of knowing you and the wonderful clan, I too, have so many great memories. Every visit was a happy time; every holiday special, filled with joy and excitement. Our children so loved our Christmas celebrations at Grandma and Grandpa's! You always made it special for us, so thank you.

We always looked forward to your visits to our home as well. It was such a wonderful time for all of us and the memories of family vacations spent together, such fun! Do you recall visiting the Hartsook, California's Gold Country and having our own personal tour guide at the California Missions? I do, and they are wonderful memories for me!

I loved being a part of such a big family and so enjoyed the stories and tales of each and every member. It was great hearing the stories of when your mother and father, along with their families, first came from the Old Country, Armenia, to the United States. Listening about their struggles to earn a living, learn a new language and how they educated themselves, so they could create a good life for their families, made me realize how blessed I am to be a part of this one, with its rich and beautiful history.

I'm sorry, Mom, for not being there to help you when you needed someone to care for and attend to your needs. I feel sad and ashamed that more wasn't done for you. No one noticed that you needed help, or how much you were suffering. You spent most of your time alone and you were slipping away from us. If I'd been with you, I could have made a difference and made life more comfortable for you. I am so sorry and wish I could turn time back and do it over.

My hope is that someday you will find comfort in knowing that some of your precious memorabilia is in our safekeeping. Your photo albums, scrapbooks, yearbooks, journals, and the love letters you and Dad wrote to one another while he was away during the war are tucked away. The letters are still neatly organized by date and lovingly tied with your pretty ribbon. We also have the hope chest you so loved and your piano sits in the loving hands of your granddaughter, who now plays. Know that we all cherish your memories and the things that meant so much to you.

I love you, Mom; we all love you. We're truly heartbroken seeing what your life has become. Our promise to you - doing our very best to see that you never suffer and that you receive the best care possible. You are in my prayers daily and my thoughts always. Again, thank you for all the wonderful memories, for which I am grateful. You are a very special person, and I'm blessed for having known you. May God bless and be with you.

Love, always and forever,

Chris - February 14, 2012

LIFE WITH LARRY

There's so much to tell, I suppose it's best to begin with how we met. Larry and I were introduced through the Couples organization at our church and we became casual friends. Although I knew his wife and one of his three sons, the relationship we shared did not extend beyond the church group. In January of 1986, his wife passed away, as did my husband. At the time, I was fifty and Larry was sixty-eight.

The following spring, a singles group started up in our church. They called it Senior Singles, which I didn't like, because I did not yet consider myself a senior. That aside, the membership was made up of a very nice group of people I had come to know over time, and attending a few of the scheduled gatherings got me out of the house. Larry was also in attendance, so we found ourselves participating in group activities together, approximately once each month.

In August of that same year, he invited me out for dinner. I had to decline, due to a previous engagement, but when he asked again, the invitation was accepted. We shared a nice dinner along the waterfront in downtown Portland, and despite the fact that it was refreshing to be out again, a part of me felt as though I was cheating on my late husband, Ed. Putting that notion away, I found it enjoyable to be able to talk about feelings with someone who had had similar experiences. There was always plenty to discuss; we often spoke for hours about our respective spouses and how it felt to lose them.

During that same dinner, I remember sharing that my husband and I had planned on taking golf lessons together, prior to his passing. The following afternoon, Larry phoned to ask if it would be too intrusive for him to stop by my home, as he had something for me. He arrived with a putter he'd found on sale in a golf shop and couldn't resist buying, hoping I would accept it. Back in the day, Larry had been a very good golfer, but by the time we got together, his game needed work. As with all golf lovers, that never deterred him, and his passion for the sport remained strong. I cherished that special putter and never considered changing it for another.

We continued to see a lot of each other, as merely good friends who loved sharing memories of family and our beloved spouses. But the day came when we labeled ourselves as "officially dating." Because I was still working, our outings were mainly in the evenings. Occasionally I'd cook, but the majority of the time, we went to restaurants. Larry was "old school" and insisted on paying, so my grocery bills definitely decreased. Traveling together was next on the agenda, beginning with a weekend jaunt to San Francisco. We stayed in separate rooms, I might add, which he insisted on taking care of. There we dined royally, at the Top of the Mark and attended a very funny play entitled "The Foreigner." And still, even though I was having a lot of fun, there was a sense of guilt gnawing at me; everything felt so surreal.

Our next trip was to Reno, which was my first experience entering a casino. Larry liked to gamble a little and I decided to try my luck at the slots, which was not profitable for me. Over the months, it seemed we were spending more and more time together. I have a fond memory of taking a drive to the coast and singing the entire way, after I bought my new car. On that same trip, we went to the theater and listened to music in the park. That is also the point in time when I was introduced to most of his family and he met several members of mine.

Larry owned a condo timeshare that could be used in a number of locations. A suggestion was made that we take advantage of the Hawaii property in the spring, so after much consideration, we each bought a ticket and started planning. As the departure date drew nearer, we came to the realization that our relationship had grown further than friendship. Our feelings for one another were so strong, we decided marriage was the next logical step. Because Larry was nearly seventy and recognizing that most likely one of us would have to endure the loss of the other down the line, we agreed that spending five years as man and wife would be a more suitable option over continuing to live apart. We planned a small wedding at our church on May 23rd, less than three weeks after the engagement.

In attendance were Larry's three sons with their wives, my sons, one of whom was in the Marines and just returning from a stint at sea, and finally my daughter, who filled the role as Matron of Honor. We considered ourselves very fortunate to have the support of our grown children. Looking back, our decision to marry must have felt a bit awkward for them, and although they spent very little time together outside of the wedding, the entire group was fairly compatible. Aside from the fact that it was Memorial Day weekend and any prior plans had to be scrapped, the focus of the day remained on us. We hadn't realized that it was a holiday weekend at the time, but there were no complaints from either family.

Following the wedding, I was back to work for one
week, then off to Kauai for a lovely honeymoon.
Once we returned, the decision was made to con-
solidate residences. We each listed our home, enabling us to buy one together. This is also the time
when Larry took over the finances, which, prior
to our marriage, had always been my responsibility. Our recurring joke was that the payment re-
cipients wouldn't know what to do when someone
paid bills as promptly as he did. To avoid getting
rusty, I occasionally pitched in and always insisted
that he keep me in the loop. Larry was a retired
CPA and in his prime, a very good one. It only
made sense that he assumed this task, as he liked
crunching numbers. In fact, he loved numbers so
much that counting everything became his ritual!
If we went up a flight of stairs, he counted the steps;
when we attended a meeting or a class, he counted
heads; in our yard, he took an on-going inventory
of the different types of flowers and shrubs we had
planted.

Yes, he spent hours working on our income projec-
tions for the coming years, only because he loved
doing it. On numerous occasions he mentioned
that we would be just fine without my income, and
should I decide to retire from my job, we would be
free to come and go as we pleased. After all, Larry
had taken that step several years prior and wanted to enjoy the present with me, so in January of
1988, I complied. Despite his retired status, he did

retain a few of his seasonal tax clients, but made certain that the work didn't interfere with his free time. Whenever changes arose in any area of our life, he never complained. His patent response was "We'll adjust it." He was always kind, thoughtful, loving, and giving to me.

Larry and I were becoming a very strong and loving team that enjoyed each other's company. We were extremely compatible and shared many fun and interesting experiences. For both of us, this was our "second life," entirely different from our prior marriages. Our first unions were very happy, but now there were so many new elements being introduced to us. Both my late husband and I were employed until his passing, which didn't afford us the time to do many of the things that I was later able to experience with Larry. One of those new elements was learning how to golf. We played a fair bit at a par-3 course nearby and for a few years, we were out there four or five times each week. From time to time, I was able to beat his score, but in all fairness, that was only because his game was rusty. Following our play, we would stop at our favorite brew pub for a bite, before returning home. Larry ordered his standard beer, a cola for me and we split a BLT. Our life was what I would call "normal."

Games were another important ritual for us. Working on puzzles, crosswords & playing board games, specifically Upwards, a three-dimensional Scrabble game, were activities that Larry and I enjoyed. Together, we sometimes played up to three rounds of that game, every day for fifteen of our twenty two years together. Our skill levels were equally matched and of course steadily improved with all the practice. I also learned to play Bridge, which led us to join a Bridge group comprised of friends from church. We remained active in our church and both served as Deacons for three years. As well, I was on the church board during that period. Larry and I also participated in a dinner club through the same group and shared in hosting an event once each year. To this day, the same individuals still meet and it is comforting; most of our social life was centered within this same bunch of friends, whom we thoroughly enjoyed.

Traveling became fairly frequent, because we could stay at Larry's timeshares. The condo units were great and we spent time in a number of them. Some of the destinations we visited were Palm Springs, Hawaii, Banff, Tahoe, Sun Valley, Yosemite, Grand Canyon, Colorado, New Mexico, Yellowstone, and Arizona. We also took cruises to Alaska and the Caribbean and traveled to England and Ireland. Larry and I had such a nice life together. Balancing holidays between families worked out well; we loved being with all of them and watching the grandchildren grow up to form lives of their own. Although the travel was exciting, home was always a welcome spot to be for both of us, and to this day I still live in that house we purchased together.

Everything I have shared so far is relevant, because it was at this juncture that I first began to notice some of the behavioral changes. The first subtle change of note was related to Larry's tax work. He began to struggle and make errors, which fortunately were caught and adjusted, but oftentimes, I had to step in and assist him. Shortly thereafter, the decision was made to discontinue working for his clients and at that point, I was in complete agreement. Regarding our personal bills, rather than pay them, he tossed them into a pile on his desk, so I quietly took over. One day he caught me writing checks and asked me what I was doing. After I responded, the issue was never brought up again.

With respect to our games, it became increasingly difficult for him to complete a crossword puzzle, and there was a very apparent deterioration with his memory. He no longer was able to beat me when we'd play our board games, and he was still aware enough to recognize when I was letting him win. In an effort to save his feelings, I suggested that we not play as often and needless to say, our games became a thing of the past. At the time, I attributed these behavioral shifts to nothing more than mere age creeping up on him. If I'm being honest, my mind won't always cooperate for me like it used to. Perhaps at that time, it was only aging, but in hindsight, it may also have been a precursor of things to come.

My husband and I had a little Dachshund named Lollie. Every day we would take her for walks together, covering the same route. One afternoon, Larry ventured out solo with our pup and was gone longer than usual. Apparently, he had strayed from the usual track and could not figure out how to get home. Fortunately, he had the presence of mind to ask for help and located our address in his wallet. I was very thankful when he returned and going forward, took care to monitor his whereabouts more closely.

Familiarity became terribly important because within his familiar surroundings, life ran a lot smoother. On occasion, if our routine changed (which never bothered him before), or we visited some new place, Larry would become confused. Other than a few jaunts to visit family, see the beach, or take a short drive, our days of exploration became non-existent. Traveling to any place unfamiliar to him now only increased his confusion. When I left to attend my son's retirement, I asked Larry's boy to stay, as I could no longer leave him alone. Again, that was presenting him with a different situation; one without me in it. He proceeded to call me every day to ask when I was returning. Approximately every five years, one of his loving sons accompanied Larry to visit his older sister out-of-state, providing me with some much needed alone time.

Recalling one day back in 2003, I arrived home from a meeting to find that the dishwasher had overflowed. He had tried to do dishes for me, but ended up putting the wrong soap in the dispenser, which resulted in a flow of suds everywhere. Realizing there was a problem, Larry grabbed a mop and bucket, but couldn't remember what to do with them. That was actually the event which expedited my decision never to leave him alone again. Going forward, when I went to the grocery store, he would walk alongside me, until it became a strain for him. Waiting in the car didn't settle well, so my solution was buying him a latte at the coffee nook and picking him up when I was done shopping. On occasion, our friends were kind enough to visit with my husband, or take him to lunch if I needed to run errands.

The behavioral changes continued to progress, and as Larry's memory decreased, it seemed that his drinking did the opposite. He was a whiskey lover and enjoyed a small glass each afternoon. There were no indications of overindulgence, but it was apparent that we were buying it more often. It was suggested to me that I fill the bottle with a bit of water to stretch it out, but my guilt got the best of me and I stopped. Shortly after, I recognized that my husband didn't notice the difference, so I resumed that practice. A similar situation presented itself when I traveled to my granddaughter's wedding and left Larry with one of his sons. Endeavoring to make his dad feel at home, his son bought a bottle of his favorite whiskey and discovered it empty in a flash. In hindsight, I wonder if his accelerated consumption was attributed to not remembering that he'd already had a drink.

On the whole, we both enjoyed good health. Outside of the minor acid reflux, or age-related arthritis, health issues were few. That is, until the summer of his 76th year. As mentioned, our traveling days were few and far between, but it was his birthday month, so we decided to visit Tahoe, Yosemite, and San Francisco. The altitude caused Larry to experience shortness of breath, and upon examination, it was determined that he had a faulty aortic valve. Once we returned home, he had the valve replaced, a pacemaker installed, and fully recovered. This juncture also marked the end of his distance driving, as his feet were occasionally going numb on the pedals and he was directionally challenged due to the memory loss.

The cognitive decline continued to accelerate, and my assistance was needed more than ever before. I specifically remember a New Year's Eve party we attended at the home of some friends. On the car ride over, Larry repeatedly asked me where we were headed and who was hosting the party. He practiced the names I furnished him, but had no recollection of their identities. This was the same group of individuals that we had entertained in our home multiple times, but he swore he had never met them.

Family became unrecognizable as well, and that included me. During a visit from his son and daughter-in-law, his goodbyes were expressed as "nice meeting you." It always seemed that he enjoyed being with the relatives, but as soon as they left, Larry would again ask me who they were and which child belonged to which family. Periodically, my husband called me by his sister's name, or he would refer to me as "Mother." I can still recall him looking at me, wondering who I was. I'd enlighten him, but it didn't register. The only thing he wanted to know was where I lived and when I was going home. One morning he got up and was wandering around the house aim- lessly. I asked him if I could do anything and he asked me to help him find his wife. "Her name is Virginia, do you know her?" In fact, one time he asked me to buy him a card to give to his bride for their anniversary.

Meal time also became a challenge, because he lacked any recall that he'd eaten. If I fixed him something, he would often take a few bites and state that he was no longer hungry. Then a short time later, he was accusing me of withholding food from him, which couldn't have been further from the truth. Another thing about my husband is that he always took care of himself and his appearance. Now, there were occasions when he'd appear at breakfast, unshaven with his trousers over his pajamas, or he'd dress in his hat and coat to come to bed - all of this, completely out of character.

Paranoia settled in, which brought about frequent hallucinations of imaginary strangers entering our home. If we were watching a game show, he asked me how much I had won; TV shows became reality. His thought patterns were jumbled, which led to his searching for toothpaste in the refrigerator, or forgetting something as simple as how to fetch a glass of water. Larry was an avid reader. I recall an instance when he had forgotten how to change his hearing aid batteries, so he opted to throw them away. He told me they were hampering his ability to read. In truth, his eyesight was suffering and it became difficult for him to see the words, but that didn't stop him. I'd still find Larry, book in hand, intently perusing the pages of some novel, but upon closer examination, I'd notice that the book was turned upside down.

Ingrained in his being was his CPA certification, and money became his focus. He developed the notion that he was responsible for the financial well-being of everyone and wanted to give away all that we had. I found myself racing to our mailbox daily to ensure the mail was picked up before Larry got there, as he wanted to donate to each and every cause. I felt terrible because in a way, it was deceitful, but I needed to protect both of us.

Several times he stated, "I think I am losing my mind," and I often wondered what it was like for him inside. Was he frightened, or did he have any sense of what was happening? My feeling is that it must have been terrible for Larry to be in that state. But, it was confusing for me as well, because there were periods of total clarity. In time though, I grew to be patient with the recognition that Larry's actions were no longer under his control. Unfortunately, the string of irrational incidences related to conduct continued to grow. It is important to note that all of the aforementioned events took place prior to his diagnosis.

We had wonderful friends who were beginning to notice the deportment changes. They were kind individuals who listened to Larry's repetitive stories with tremendous patience and not a murmur of "I've heard that before." Talking to his sons was uncomfortable for me. Because they lived some distance from us, they weren't experiencing what I was day-to-day and they questioned my evaluation. Larry's "war stories" were enjoyable to hear, but they had no idea how often he actually shared the same tales. The boys were great conversationalists and their father was a good listener, so it went unnoticed that due to the short term memory failing, he had little to lend. At this point, the story "crafting" came into play.

He told them about a trip he took to Antarctica; another time, while on a Mediterranean cruise the captain of the ship supposedly let Larry off in the Holy Land and he walked the entire length of that land. The stories had substance and were very believable; however, they were not true. When it came to events that truly did take place, his timelines were in disarray. There was no point in trying to correct him, or explain that it didn't happen. I learned early on that one cannot win an argument with an Alzheimer's victim. (At that time, he still hadn't been officially diagnosed, but I had my suspicions.) You learn that little white lies have their place, or just say you agree and continue doing things your own way. Even though deception didn't feel right, I knew not to beat myself up. Sometimes, that was the only way to handle situations, and Larry would have no recollection of it, anyway.

I finally spoke to his doctor about the problem, but he dismissed my concerns, attributing the behaviors to the aging process. Nevertheless, I knew there was something more. Refusing to give up, I made an appointment with another physician, and prior to the visit, sent him a long letter outlining my concerns. He was very kind and took me seriously, immediately referring us to a neurologist, who diagnosed the Alzheimer's. This came as no surprise to me and was a welcome verification of what I had already suspected. The doctor explained that the disease would plateau and dip, similar to stairs. There could be prolonged periods of clarity, but the situation would never improve. Medicine could aid in slowing the progression; however, the outcome was inevitable.

Shortly thereafter, I began taking Larry to an Adult Day Care center, once each week. This provided me with a few hours to run errands and they really flew by. Larry balked at going every time, but they did fuss over him and he liked the attention. Somehow he had the idea that it was work I was taking him to, so he had no interest. But I told him they really needed his help with the other people. Another suggestion from family and friends was to join a support group. Taking their advice, I did begin attending a group, which met monthly, and I met some very nice people. Also offered through this group was a course on taking care of oneself as a caregiver, which was very helpful. There were staff members around, so I was able to take my husband

1 of1 of ...

with me, although he didn't understand why needed this class, because in his mind, he wa. fine. Journaling was a great release for me, as well, during his progression. Each night at bedtime, I would jot down the events of the day to clear my head. Some of the occurrences were so bizarre, it was great to have a record of them. One can't make this stuff up!

Health challenges began to present themselves to Larry. In addition to Alzheimer's, he had developed congestive heart disease and his blood pressure was acting up. He'd become less steady on his feet and was experiencing quite a few falls, with one resulting in a hospital stay due to a brain bleed. Any semblance of table manners had vanished, he began sleeping more, and no longer knew how to dress, shower, or brush his own teeth. Everything I did appeared to irritate him, and he didn't hesitate to let me know it. A good deal of the time, his speech had turned to gibberish, and when I was not able to decipher his words, he became extremely frustrated. A request was made to label everything for him, including family photos, with the hope that doing so would help to aid his memory. Sadly, it did not. Within a short period of time, his depression, frustration and anger had risen to a level that exceeded my patience threshold. Phoning his doctor, I was told to administer an anti-psychotic medicine and then bring him in the next day. By the following morning, he

✓   .ly catatonic, and getting him to the
             without help was no easy task. He re-
          unresponsive during the appointment,
        . doctor admitted him to the hospital.

.y husband's sons arrived the next morning to be
with their dad. Out of his comfort zone, Larry became even more confused and wanted to return
home. His doctor declared to the family that it
was time to find a facility where he could receive
around-the-clock care. Although I knew it was
coming, I don't think you are ever fully prepared.
It was a major step for all of us, but the entire
group agreed it was in Larry's best interest. After
touring several facilities and listening about their
programs, we chose a residence near our home.
We were fortunate that they had a vacancy, and
to promote a smooth transition, the doctor kept
Larry in the hospital, while we were making the
arrangements. In January of 2008, Larry's sons
drove him to his new home at the Senior Living
Facility. Endeavoring to make his environment appear as familiar as possible, we had brought over a
number of his possessions, but I'll never be certain
if it made a difference. That day was one of my
darkest, and his boys were also heartbroken.

I harbored plenty of guilt for quite some time over
our decision. Many tears were shed and there was
a lot of second guessing. The transition was difficult for everyone, especially Larry. All familiarity

had vanished, and he didn't know where he was or why he couldn't go to our "nice house." Long before, he had made me promise that under no circumstances would I put him into "one of those places." My response was that we had no way of knowing what our needs might be in the future, so I couldn't make that promise.

The staff at his residence was kind and took care to treat each patient in a dignified manner, irrespective of his or her condition. It was mostly comprised of young women, but there were a few male employees. When bath time rolled around, Larry refused to let "the little girls" help him shower (Can't say I blame him), but there was one mature caregiver who was occasionally able to break through his stubborn streak.

Eating was a problem, which wasn't new, as his appetite had been decreasing for some time. I made a point of visiting him every day in the beginning, right around lunch time, when I could encourage him to eat. His favorites were corn cereal and hamburgers, so, if he wouldn't eat what was served, they made sure he got what he liked. Because these types of environments are sedentary, water consumption is vital in staving off urinary tract infections, or UTIs. Larry wasn't a water fan, but they addressed that by bringing him his coffee. All-in-all, they took good care of him.

Larry's room was in the secured area called The Cottage, and it was filled with people in various stages of Alzheimer's, Parkinson's, and other diseases with similar symptoms. It was designed with a home-like feel to make the residents as comfortable as possible. Every day, the inhabitants were dressed and brought out to the hub to be together. This consisted of a small kitchen area where freshly baked goods were made daily (the aroma was wonderful). The building also offered one sitting area with a TV and another which overlooked a courtyard. A communal dining room was where family-style meals were served and it was very pleasant. Each afternoon they hosted Tea Time for those who wished to partake. Guests were always welcome and I often stayed around to participate. His boys visited as often as they could manage, but like many others, they found their dad's situation challenging. Often, they took him for a drive, or coffee, and it was a nice change of pace to get Larry out in the fresh air. On several occasions one of Larry's boys brought his little daughter over to visit. Spending time with his granddaughter always brightened the day for my husband, as well as the other Cottage residents.

When summer arrived, my husband and I sat on the patio together, where I attempted to read to him. That effort was short-lived, as he could not understand the story line. Periodically, he asked if he could go home with me, or come and live at my house. It broke my heart. Even though he didn't always recognize me when I came, his face always would light up the moment he saw me. I found it difficult when it was time to leave, so for a while, I would simply sneak out once he fell asleep. Somehow he figured that out and told me he wasn't going to sleep anymore, because I wouldn't be there when he woke up. You just never knew when he would be cognizant, or not.

In any facility it's challenging to keep track of personal belongings, especially on laundry day. Because of that, I took his clothes home every day and washed them myself. Plenty of other items went missing, because, due to the mental decline, people no longer had the capability of understanding boundaries. I'm the one who needed to adjust and simply be thankful that the man I loved was clean and cared for. After all, in the big scheme of things, the "stuff" wasn't important.

Eventually, Larry lost his interest in the outside world. He became very impatient, was losing weight and looking frail. Incidents of falling became more frequent, but he didn't like to use the walker. His friends stopped visiting, as it was too difficult for them to witness the decline. It just seemed like my husband was beginning to shut down. A recommendation was made for hospice to get involved. These individuals are wonderfully caring and compassionate. Right away, Larry was taken off of the majority of his medications, provided a wheelchair when the time came, and any other medical supplies that were required. Hospice also took over monitoring his vitals, bathing, etc. There were times, however, that I would arrive to find that the staff hadn't gotten him up, or he was lying in bed without covers. Their job is difficult, but it is easy to become complacent when the patient can't voice his needs. Instances when more than one patient needs extra care, or when several are having a bad day, probably come up more often than not, I get it. But, when you are paying that exorbitant monthly rate to have your loved one taken care of, you expect more. That is precisely why I feel advocacy is so important. Soon I made sure to arrive at a variety of times throughout the day, unannounced.

On Father's Day, one month before Larry died, his son came to visit and handed him a greeting card. My husband began to eat it, along with chewing the table cloth and doing other nonsensical things. It was truly difficult for anyone to witness, especially his poor boy. Within weeks, Larry was bedridden and deteriorating steadily. He no longer wished to be moved, and I believe a mere touch was painful for him, due to his frailty. More than once, we believed the end was near, but each time he rallied. Both sides of the family took turns spending time with him and saying their goodbyes. The staff was very caring, kind, and there for me throughout this period.

I've been told that hearing is the last sense to go and that people can comprehend what is being said, even if they're unable to respond. Keeping that in mind, we talked strictly about good times and happy memories. In my belief, there comes a moment when a person is straddling two worlds, the "present" and the "next dimension." Well, I witnessed that happening with my husband. In the back of my mind, there was also a concern that Larry would pass away on my birthday and leave me holding that memory forever; he held on until after.

Some may never understand me when I say that it was a relief to all of us when Larry took his last breath. Throughout the life of this ordeal, we had all experienced an abundance of pain and sadness, as that mind-stealing disease took away the man we knew and loved. It's incredibly sad to me, because the afflicted have no chance of improving, and, as such, the indignities associated with this disease become a part of those individuals, transforming their lives into ones they would not have chosen.

Outside of sharing these memories, I continue to focus on the good times and want to emphasize that there were many of those! Disease-related changes came about gradually over the years and although at times life became challenging, there was never a question about the existence of an enduring love between us. I'm very grateful that I was able to be there for Larry, and my only regret is that this had to happen at all.

Virginia

ABOUT THE AUTHOR

"Perspective is an incredibly powerful tool. It tempers how we receive information, and guides what we choose do with it."

Writing "Where's My Purse" has been a challenging exercise, due to the sensitive nature of the content. At times I have struggled with the notion that some may perceive me as "insensitive," which I am not. Looking at select situations with a comedic eye helps ME cope, and that's how my mom would want it. I was raised in a home where laughter was used as a defense mechanism, a vehicle for communication and our pharmaceutical of choice. When we learned that Mom had Alzheimer's, I found myself drowning in a sea of self-pity, yet JoAnn was the one who drew the short straw. In other words, I was making it about me. The only obvious solution was to change MY perspective. Once that adjustment was made, I became a highly effective advocate for her and found peace.

There's also the little matter of opening up my private world to total strangers; very uncharacteristic of me. But, I understand how it feels to walk this road with someone you love and feel helpless. Granted, there's an abundance of reference material just waiting to be downloaded, but what I have valued more during this process, is hearing from others in similar situations, which has validated my feelings.

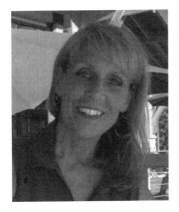

T.A. Sorensen resides in the Pacific Northwest with her husband, where she works as a designer. After spending two years in Colorado and twelve years in Toronto, Canada, they returned to be closer to her family in her beautiful birthplace.

"You will never experience personal growth, if you fear taking chances. And, you will never become successful, if you operate without integrity."

WHERE'S MY PURSE?

T. A. SORENSEN

12518996R00109

Made in the USA
San Bernardino, CA
19 June 2014